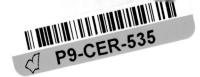
Virtual Clinical Excursions—Psychiatric

for

Varcarolis and Halter:
Foundations of Psychiatric Mental Health Nursing,
6th Edition

prepared by

Susan Fertig McDonald, DNP, RN, CS
Clinical Nurse Specialist—Psychiatry
VA San Diego Healthcare System
San Diego, California

software developed by

Wolfsong Informatics, LLC
Tucson, Arizona

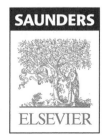

SAUNDERS

ELSEVIER

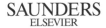

3251 Riverport Lane
Maryland Heights, Missouri 63043

VIRTUAL CLINICAL EXCURSIONS—PSYCHIATRIC FOR   ISBN: 978-1-4377-1524-8
VARCAROLIS AND HALTER:
FOUNDATIONS OF PSYCHIATRIC MENTAL HEALTH NURSING
SIXTH EDITION
Copyright © 2010, 2006 by Saunders, an imprint of Elsevier Inc.

Although for mechanical reasons all pages of this publication are perforated, only those pages
imprinted with an Elsevier Inc. copyright notice are intended for removal.

Notice

Knowledge and best practice in this field are constantly changing. As new research and experience
broaden our knowledge, changes in practice, treatment and drug therapy may become necessary or
appropriate. Readers are advised to check the most current information provided (i) on procedures
featured or (ii) by the manufacturer of each product to be administered, to verify the recommended
dose or formula, the method and duration of administration, and contraindications. It is the
responsibility of the practitioner, relying on their own experience and knowledge of the patient, to
make diagnoses, to determine dosages and the best treatment for each individual patient, and to
take all appropriate safety precautions. To the fullest extent of the law, neither the Publisher nor
the Authors assumes any liability for any injury and/or damage to persons or property arising out
or related to any use of the material contained in this book.

ISBN: 978-1-4377-1524-8

Editor: *Jeff Downing*
Associate Developmental Editor: *Krissy Prysmiki*
Project Manager: *Tracey Schriefer*
Book Production Manager: *Gayle May*

Printed in the United States of America

Last digit is the print number: 9 8 7 6 5 4

Workbook
prepared by

Susan Fertig McDonald, DNP, RN, CS
Clinical Nurse Specialist—Psychiatry
VA San Diego Healthcare System
San Diego, California

Textbook

Elizabeth M. Varcarolis, RN, MA
Professor Emeritus
Formerly Duty Chairperson, Department of Nursing
Burough of Manhattan Community College
New York, New York

Associate Fellow
Albert Ellis Institute for Rational Emotional Behavior Therapy (REBT)
New York, New York

Margaret J. Halter, PhD, PMHCNS-BC
Associate Professor
College of Nursing
University of Akron
Akron, Ohio

Reviewer

Carissa Enright, MSN, RN
Clinical Assistant Professor
Nursing Faculty, College of Nursing
Texas Woman's University
Dallas, Texas

Contents

Table of Contents
Varcarolis and Halter:
Foundations of Psychiatric Mental Health Nursing, 6th Edition

Unit 6—Interventions for Special Populations

Unit 7—Other Intervention Modalities

Getting Started

GETTING SET UP

■ **MINIMUM SYSTEM REQUIREMENTS**

WINDOWS®

Windows Vista®, XP, 2000 (Recommend Windows XP/2000)
Pentium® III processor (or equivalent) @ 600 MHz (Recommend 800 MHz or better)
256 MB of RAM (Recommend 1 GB or more for Windows Vista)
800 x 600 screen size (Recommend 1024 x 768)
Thousands of colors
12x CD-ROM drive

Note: Windows Vista and XP require administrator privileges for installation.

MACINTOSH® (*Note:* This CD will not work in Mac Lion 10.7)

MAC OS X (up to 10.6)
Apple Power PC G3 @ 500 MHz or better
128 MB of RAM (Recommend 256 MB or more)
800 x 600 screen size (Recommend 1024 x 768)
Thousands of colors
12x CD-ROM drive
Stereo speakers or headphones

■ INSTALLATION INSTRUCTIONS

WINDOWS

1. Insert the *Virtual Clinical Excursions—Psychiatric* CD-ROM.
2. The setup screen should appear automatically if the current product is not already installed. Windows Vista users may be asked to authorize additional security prompts.
3. Follow the onscreen instructions during the setup process.

   If the setup screen does *not* appear automatically (and *Virtual Clinical Excursions—Psychiatric* has not been installed already):
   a. Click the **My Computer** icon on your desktop or on your Start menu.
   b. Double-click on your CD-ROM drive.
   c. If installation does not start at this point:
      (1) Click the **Start** icon on the taskbar and select the **Run** option.
      (2) Type d:\setup.exe (where "d:\" is your CD-ROM drive) and press **OK**.
      (3) Follow the onscreen instructions for installation.

MACINTOSH

1. Insert the *Virtual Clinical Excursions—Psychiatric* CD in the CD-ROM drive. The disk icon will appear on your desktop.

2. Double-click on the disk icon.

3. Double-click on the VCEPSYCH_MAC run file.

Note: Virtual Clinical Excursions—Psychiatric for Macintosh does not have an installation setup and can only be run directly from the CD.

■ HOW TO USE VIRTUAL CLINICAL EXCURSIONS—PSYCHIATRIC

WINDOWS

1. Double-click on the *Virtual Clinical Excursions—Psychiatric* icon located on your desktop.
2. Or navigate to the program via the Windows Start menu.

Note: If your computer uses Windows Vista, right-click on the desktop shortcut and choose **Properties**. In the Compatability Mode, check the box for "Run as Administrator." Below is a screen capture to show what this looks like.

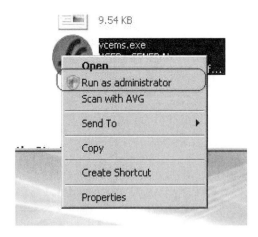

MACINTOSH

1. Insert the *Virtual Clinical Excursions—Psychiatric* CD in the CD-ROM drive. The disk icon will appear on your desktop.

2. Double-click on the disk icon.

3. Double-click on the VCEPSYCH_MAC run file.

SCREEN SETTINGS

For best results, your computer monitor resolution should be set at a minimum of 800 x 600. The number of colors displayed should be set to "thousands or higher" (High Color or 16 bit) or "millions of colors" (True Color or 24 bit).

Windows

1. From the **Start** menu, select **Control Panel** (on some systems, you will first go to **Settings**, then to **Control Panel**).
2. Double-click on the **Display** icon.
3. Click on the **Settings** tab.
4. Under **Screen resolution** use the slider bar to select **800 by 600 pixels**.
5. Access the **Colors** drop-down menu by clicking on the down arrow.
6. Select **High Color (16 bit)** or **True Color (24 bit)**.
7. Click on **OK**.
8. You may be asked to verify the setting changes. Click **Yes**.
9. You may be asked to restart your computer to accept the changes. Click **Yes**.

Macintosh

1. Select the **Monitors** control panel.
2. Select **800 x 600** (or similar) from the **Resolution** area.
3. Select **Thousands** or **Millions** from the **Color Depth** area.

WEB BROWSERS

Supported web browsers include Microsoft Internet Explorer (IE) version 7.0 or higher and Mozilla 3.0 or higher.

If you use America Online® (AOL) for web access, you will need AOL version 4.0 or higher and one of the browsers listed above. Do not use earlier versions of AOL with earlier versions of IE, because you will have difficulty accessing many features.

For best results with AOL:
- Connect to the Internet using AOL version 4.0 or higher.
- Open a private chat within AOL (this allows the AOL client to remain open, without asking whether you wish to disconnect while minimized).
- Minimize AOL.
- Launch a recommended browser.

■ **TECHNICAL SUPPORT**

Technical support for this product is available 24 hours a day, seven days a week, excluding holidays. Before calling, be sure that your computer meets the minimum system requirements to run this software. Inside the United States and Canada, call 1-800-222-9570. Outside North America, call 314-447-8094. You may also fax your questions to 314-447-8078 or contact Technical Support through e-mail: technical.support@elsevier.com.

Trademarks: Windows, Macintosh, Pentium, and America Online are registered trademarks.

ACCESSING *Virtual Clinical Excursions—Psychiatric* FROM EVOLVE

The product you have purchased is part of the Evolve family of online courses and learning resources. Please read the following information thoroughly to get started.

To access your instructor's course on Evolve:

Your instructor will provide you with the username and password needed to access this specific course on the Evolve Learning System. Once you have received this information, please follow these instructions:

1. Go to the Evolve student page (http://evolve.elsevier.com/student).

2. Enter your username and password in the **Login to My Evolve** area and click the **Login** button.

3. You will be taken to your personalized **My Evolve** page, where the course will be listed in the **My Courses** module.

TECHNICAL REQUIREMENTS

To use an Evolve course, you will need access to a computer that is connected to the Internet and equipped with web browser software that supports frames. For optimal performance, it is recommended that you have speakers and use a high-speed Internet connection. However, slower dial-up modems (56 K minimum) are acceptable.

Whichever browser you use, the browser preferences must be set to enable cookies and the cache must be set to reload every time.

Enable Cookies

Browser	Steps
Internet Explorer (IE) 7.0 or higher	1. Select **Tools → Internet Options**. 2. Select **Privacy** tab. 3. Use the slider (slide down) to **Accept All Cookies**. 4. Click **OK**. -OR- 3. Click the **Advanced** button. 4. Click the check box next to **Override Automatic Cookie Handling**. 5. Click the **Accept** radio buttons under **First-party Cookies** and **Third-party Cookies**. 6. Click **OK**.
Mozilla Firefox 3.0 or higher	1. Select **Tools → Options**. 2. Select the **Privacy** icon. 3. Click to expand Cookies. 4. Select **Allow sites to set cookies**. 5. Click **OK**.

Set Cache to Always Reload a Page

Browser	Steps
Internet Explorer (IE) 7.0 or higher	1. Select **Tools → Internet Options**. 2. Select **General** tab. 3. Go to the **Temporary Internet Files** and click the **Settings** button. 4. Select the radio button for **Every visit to the page** and click **OK** when complete.
Mozilla Firefox 3.0 or higher	1. Select **Tools → Options**. 2. Select the **Privacy** icon. 3. Click to expand Cache. 4. Set the value to "**0**" in the **Use up to: __ MB of disk space for the cache** field. 5. Click **OK**.

Plug-Ins

Adobe Acrobat Reader—With the free Acrobat Reader software, you can view and print Adobe PDF files. Many Evolve products offer student and instructor manuals, checklists, and more in this format!

Download at: http://www.adobe.com

Apple QuickTime—Install this to hear word pronunciations, heart and lung sounds, and many other helpful audio clips within Evolve Online Courses!

Download at: http://www.apple.com

Adobe Flash Player—This player will enhance your viewing of many Evolve web pages, as well as educational short-form to long-form animation within the Evolve Learning System!

Download at: http://www.adobe.com

Adobe Shockwave Player—Shockwave is best for viewing the many interactive learning activities within Evolve Online Courses!

Download at: http://www.adobe.com

Microsoft Word Viewer—With this viewer, Microsoft Word users can share documents with those who don't have Word, and users without Word can open and view Word documents. Many Evolve products have testbank, student and instructor manuals, and other documents available for downloading and viewing on your own computer!

Download at: http://www.microsoft.com

Microsoft PowerPoint Viewer—With this viewer, you can access PowerPoint 97, 2000, and 2002 presentations even if you don't have PowerPoint. Many Evolve products have slides available for downloading and viewing on your own computer!

Download at: http://www.microsoft.com

SUPPORT INFORMATION

Live phone support is available to customers in the United States and Canada at **800-222-9570** 24 hours a day, seven days a week. Support is also available through email at technical.support@elsevier.com.

Online 24/7 support can be accessed on the Evolve website (http://evolve.elsevier.com). Resources include:

- Guided tours
- Tutorials
- Frequently asked questions (FAQs)
- Online copies of course user guides
- And much more!

A QUICK TOUR

Welcome to *Virtual Clinical Excursions—Psychiatric*, a virtual hospital setting in which you can work with multiple complex patient simulations and also learn to access and evaluate the information resources that are essential for high-quality patient care. The virtual hospital, Pacific View Regional Hospital, has realistic architecture and access to patient rooms, a Nurses' Station, and a Medication Room.

■ BEFORE YOU START

Make sure you have your textbook nearby when you use the *Virtual Clinical Excursions—Psychiatric* CD. You will want to consult topic areas in your textbook frequently while working with the CD and using this workbook.

■ HOW TO SIGN IN

- Enter your name on the Student Nurse identification badge.
- Next, click the down arrow next to **Select Floor**. This drop-down menu lists only the floors on which there are currently patients with psychiatric nursing needs: Medical-Surgical, Obstetrics, Pediatrics, and Skilled Nursing. (For this quick tour, choose **Obstetrics**.)
- Now choose one of the four periods of care in which to work. In Periods of Care 1 through 3, you can actively engage in patient assessment, entry of data in the electronic patient record (EPR), and medication administration. Period of Care 4 presents the day in review. Highlight and click the appropriate period of care. (For this quick tour, choose **Period of Care 1: 0730-0815**.)
- Click **Go**. This takes you to the Patient List screen (see example on page 11). Note that the virtual time is provided in the box at the lower left corner of the screen (0730, since we chose Period of Care 1).

Note: If you choose to work during Period of Care 4: 1900-2000, the Patient List screen is skipped since you are not able to visit patients or administer medications during the shift. Instead, you are taken directly to the Nurses' Station, where the records of all the patients on the floor are available for your review.

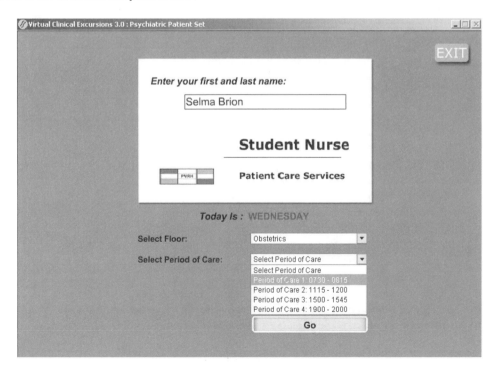

■ **PATIENT LIST**

OBSTETRICS UNIT

Dorothy Grant (Room 201)
30-week intrauterine pregnancy—A 25-year-old Caucasian multipara admitted with abdominal trauma following a domestic violence incident. Her complications include preterm labor and extensive social issues such as acquiring safe housing for her family upon discharge.

Kelly Brady (Room 203)
26-week intrauterine pregnancy—A 35-year-old Caucasian primigravida urgently admitted for progressive symptoms of preeclampsia. A history of inadequate coping with major life stressors leave her at risk for a recurrence of depression as she faces a diagnosis of HELLP syndrome and the delivery of a severely premature infant.

Laura Wilson (Room 206)
37-week intrauterine pregnancy—An 18-year-old Caucasian primigravida urgently admitted after being found unconscious. Her complications include HIV-positive status and chronic poly-substance abuse. Unrealistic expectations of parenthood and living with a chronic illness, combined with strained family relations, prompt comprehensive social and psychiatric evaluations initiated on the day of simulation.

PEDIATRIC UNIT

Tiffany Sheldon (Room 305)
Anorexia nervosa—A 14-year-old Caucasian female admitted for dehydration, electrolyte imbalance, and malnutrition following a syncope episode at home. This patient has a history of eating disorders that have required multiple hospital admissions and have strained family dynamics between mother and daughter.

MEDICAL-SURGICAL UNIT

Harry George (Room 401)
Osteomyelitis—A 54-year-old Caucasian male admitted from a homeless shelter with an infected leg. He has complications of type 2 diabetes mellitus, alcohol abuse, nicotine addiction, poor pain control, and complex psychosocial issues.

Jacquline Catanazaro (Room 402)
Asthma—A 45-year-old Caucasian female admitted with an acute asthma exacerbation and suspected pneumonia. She has complications of chronic schizophrenia, noncompliance with medication therapy, obesity, and herniated disk.

SKILLED NURSING UNIT

Kathryn Doyle (Room 503)
Rehabilitation post left hip replacement—A 79-year-old Caucasian female admitted following a complicated recovery from an ORIF. She is experiencing symptoms of malnutrition and depression due to unstable family dynamics, placing her at risk for elder abuse.

Carlos Reyes (Room 504)
Rehabilitation status post myocardial infarction—An 81-year-old Hispanic male admitted for evaluation of the need for long-term care following an acute care hospital stay. Recent cognitive changes and a diagnosis of anxiety disorder contribute to stressful family dynamics and caregiver strain.

■ HOW TO SELECT A PATIENT

- You can choose one or more patients to work with from the Patient List by checking the box to the left of the patient name(s). For this quick tour, select Dorothy Grant. (In order to receive a scorecard for a patient, the patient must be selected before proceeding to the Nurses' Station.)
- Click on **Get Report** to the right of the medical records number (MRN) to view a summary of the patient's care during the 12-hour period before your arrival on the unit.
- After reviewing the report, click on **Go to Nurses' Station** in the right lower corner to begin your care. (*Note:* If you have been assigned to care for multiple patients, you can click on **Return to Patient List** to select and review the report for each additional patient before going to the Nurses' Station.)

Note: Even though the Patient List is initially skipped when you sign in to work for Period of Care 4, you can still access this screen if you wish to review the shift report for any of the patients. To do so, simply click on **Patient List** near the top left corner of the Nurses' Station (or click on the clipboard to the left of the Kardex). Then click on **Get Report** for the patient(s) whose care you are reviewing. This may be done during any period of care.

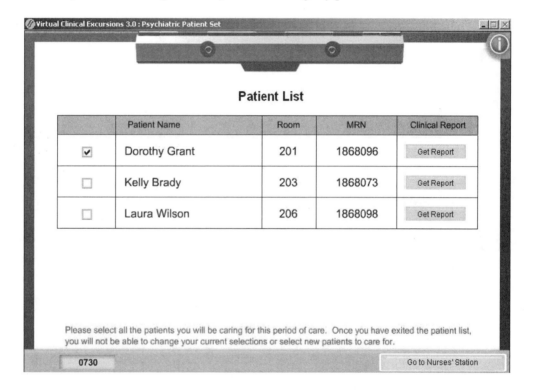

■ HOW TO FIND A PATIENT'S RECORDS

NURSES' STATION

Within the Nurses' Station, you will see:

1. A clipboard that contains the patient list for that floor.
2. A chart rack with patient charts labeled by room number, a notebook labeled Kardex, and a notebook labeled MAR (Medication Administration Record).
3. A desktop computer with access to the Electronic Patient Record (EPR).
4. A tool bar across the top of the screen that can also be used to access the Patient List, EPR, Chart, MAR, and Kardex. This tool bar is also accessible from each patient's room.
5. A Drug Guide containing information about the medications you are able to administer to your patients.
6. A tool bar across the bottom of the screen that can be used to access the Floor Map, patient rooms, Medication Room, and Drug Guide.

As you run your cursor over an item, it will be highlighted. To select, simply double-click on the item. As you use these resources, you will always be able to return to the Nurses' Station by clicking on the **Return to Nurses' Station** bar located in the right lower corner of your screen.

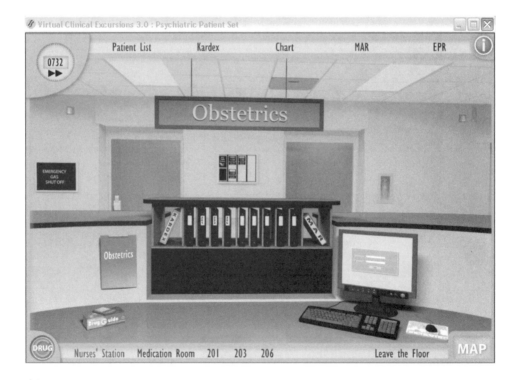

MEDICATION ADMINISTRATION RECORD (MAR)

The MAR icon located on the tool bar at the top of your screen accesses current 24-hour medications for each patient. Click on the icon and the MAR will open. (*Note:* You can also access the MAR by clicking on the MAR notebook on the far right side of the book rack in the center of the screen.) Within the MAR, tabs on the right side of the screen allow you to select patients by room number. Be careful to make sure you select the correct tab number for *your* patient rather than simply reading the first record that appears after the MAR opens. Each MAR sheet lists the following:

- Medications
- Route and dosage of each medication
- Times of administration of each medication

Note: The MAR changes each day. Expired MARs are stored in the patients' charts.

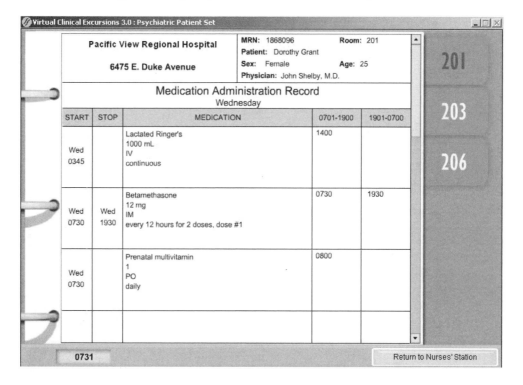

CHARTS

To access patient charts, either click on the **Chart** icon at the top of your screen or anywhere within the chart rack in the center of the Nurses' Station screen. When the close-up view appears, the individual charts are labeled by room number. To open a chart, click on the room number of the patient whose chart you wish to review. The patient's name and allergies will appear on the left side of the screen, along with a list of tabs on the right side of the screen, allowing you to view the following data:

- Allergies
- Physician's Orders
- Physician's Notes
- Nurse's Notes
- Laboratory Reports
- Diagnostic Reports
- Surgical Reports
- Consultations

- Patient Education
- History and Physical
- Nursing Admission
- Expired MARs
- Consents
- Mental Health
- Admissions
- Emergency Department

Information appears in real time. The entries are in reverse chronologic order, so use the down arrow at the right side of each chart page to scroll down to view previous entries. Flip from tab to tab to view multiple data fields or click on **Return to Nurses' Station** in the lower right corner of the screen to exit the chart.

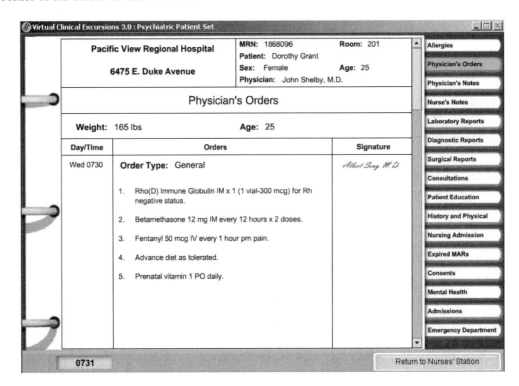

ELECTRONIC PATIENT RECORD (EPR)

The EPR can be accessed from the computer in the Nurses' Station or from the EPR icon located in the tool bar at the top of your screen. To access a patient's EPR:
- Click on either the computer screen or the **EPR** icon.
- Your username and password are automatically filled in.
- Click on **Login** to enter the EPR.
- *Note:* Like the MAR, the EPR is arranged numerically. Thus when you enter, you are initially shown the records of the patient in the lowest room number on the floor. To view the correct data for *your* patient, remember to select the correct room number, using the drop-down menu for the Patient field at the top left corner of the screen.

The EPR used in Pacific View Regional Hospital represents a composite of commercial versions being used in hospitals. You can access the EPR:
- to review existing data for a patient (by room number).
- to enter data you collect while working with a patient.

The EPR is updated daily, so no matter what day or part of a shift you are working, there will be a current EPR with the patient's data from the past days of the current hospital stay. This type of simulated EPR allows you to examine how data for different attributes have changed over time, as well as to examine data for all of a patient's attributes at a particular time. The EPR is fully functional (as it is in a real-life hospital). You can enter such data as blood pressure, breath sounds, and certain treatments. The EPR will not, however, allow you to enter data for a previous time period. Use the arrows at the bottom of the screen to move forward and backward in time.

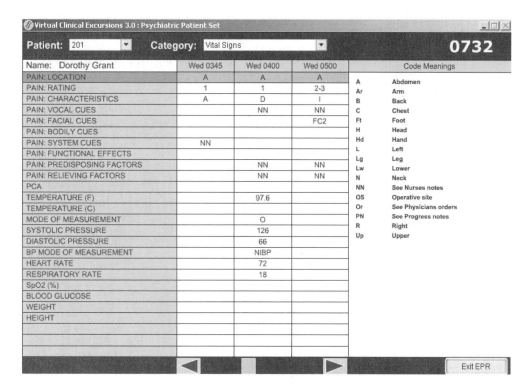

At the top of the EPR screen, you can choose patients by their room numbers. In addition, you have access to 17 different categories of patient data. To change patients or data categories, click the down arrow to the right of the room number or category.

The categories of patient data in the EPR as as follows:

- Vital Signs
- Respiratory
- Cardiovascular
- Neurologic
- Gastrointestinal
- Excretory
- Musculoskeletal
- Integumentary
- Reproductive
- Psychosocial
- Wounds and Drains
- Activity
- Hygiene and Comfort
- Safety
- Nutrition
- IV
- Intake and Output

Remember, each hospital selects its own codes. The codes used in the EPR at Pacific View Regional Hospital may be different from ones you have seen in your clinical rotations. Take some time to acquaint yourself with the codes. Within the Vital Signs category, click on any item in the left column (e.g., Pain: Characteristics). In the far-right column, you will see a list of code meanings for the possible findings and/or descriptors for that assessment area.

You will use the codes to record the data you collect as you work with patients. Click on the box in the last time column to the right of any item and wait for the code meanings applicable to that entry to appear. Select the appropriate code to describe your assessment findings and type it in the box. (*Note:* If no cursor appears within the box, click on the box again until the blue shading disappears and the blinking cursor appears.) Once the data are typed in this box, they are entered into the patient's record for this period of care only.

To leave the EPR, click on **Exit EPR** in the bottom right corner of the screen.

■ VISITING A PATIENT

From the Nurses' Station, click on the room number of the patient you wish to visit (in the tool bar at the bottom of your screen). Once you are inside the room, you will see a still photo of your patient in the top left corner. To verify that this is the correct patient, click on the **Check Armband** icon to the right of the photo. The patient's identification data will appear. If you click on **Check Allergies** (the next icon to the right), a list of the patient's allergies (if any) will replace the photo.

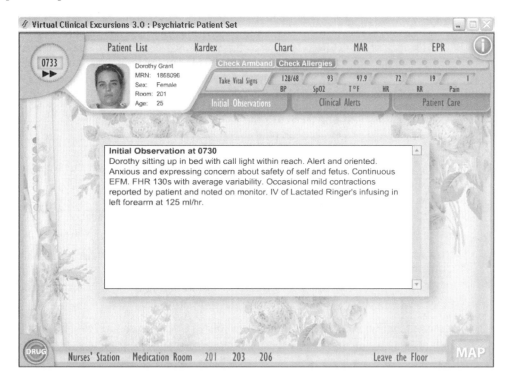

Also located in the patient's room are multiple icons you can use to assess the patient or the patient's medications. A virtual clock is provided in the upper left corner of the room to monitor your progress in real time. (*Note:* The fast-forward icon within the virtual clock will advance the time by 2-minute intervals when clicked.)

- The tool bar across the top of the screen allows you to check the **Patient List**, access the **EPR** to check or enter data, and view the patient's **Chart**, **MAR**, or **Kardex**.

- The **Take Vital Signs** icon allows you to measure the patient's up-to-the-minute blood pressure, oxygen saturation, temperature, heart rate, respiratory rate, and pain level.

- Each time you enter a patient's room, you are given an Initial Observation report to review (in the text box under the patient's photo). These notes are provided to give you a "look" at the patient as if you had just stepped into the room. You can also click on the **Initial Observations** icon to return to this box from other views within the patient's room. To the right of this icon is **Clinical Alerts**, a resource that allows you to make decisions about priority medication interventions based on emerging data collected in real time. Check this screen throughout your period of care to avoid missing critical information related to recently ordered or STAT medications.

- Clicking on **Patient Care** opens up three specific learning environments within the patient room: **Physical Assessment**, **Nurse-Client Interactions**, and **Medication Administration**.

- To perform a **Physical Assessment**, choose a body area (such as **Head & Neck**) from the column of yellow buttons. This activates a list of system subcategories for that body area (e.g., see **Sensory**, **Neurologic**, etc. in the green boxes). After you select the system you wish to evaluate, a brief description of the assessment findings will appear in a box to the right. A still photo provides a "snapshot" of how an assessment of this area might be done or what the finding might look like. For every body area, you can also click on **Equipment** on the right side of the screen.

- To the right of the Physical Assessment icon is **Nurse-Client Interactions**. Clicking on this icon will reveal the times and titles of any videos available for viewing. (*Note:* If the video you wish to see is not listed, this means you have not yet reached the correct virtual time to view that video. Check the virtual clock; you may return to access the video once its designated time has occurred—as long as you do so within the same period of care. Or you can click on the fast-forward icon within the virtual clock to advance the time by 2-minute intervals. You will then need to click again on **Patient Care** and **Nurse-Client Interactions** to refresh the screen.) To view a listed video, click on the white arrow to the right of the video title. Use the control buttons below the video to start, stop, pause, rewind, or fast-forward the action or to mute the sound.

- **Medication Administration** is the pathway that allows you to review and administer medications to a patient after you have prepared them in the Medication Room. This process is addressed further in the *How to Prepare Medications* section (pages 19-20) and in *Medications* (pages 26-30). For additional hands-on practice, see *Reducing Medication Errors* (pages 37-41).

■ HOW TO QUIT, CHANGE PATIENTS, CHANGE FLOORS, OR CHANGE PERIODS OF CARE

How to Quit: From most screens, you may click the **Leave the Floor** icon on the bottom tool bar to the right of the patient room numbers. (*Note:* From some screens, you will first need to click an **Exit** button or **Return to Nurses' Station** before clicking **Leave the Floor**.) When the Floor Menu appears, click **Exit** to leave the program.

How to Change Patients, Floors, or Periods of Care: To change patients, simply click on the new patient's room number. (You cannot receive a scorecard for a new patient, however, unless you have already selected that patient on the Patient List screen.) To change to a new period of care, to change floors, or to restart the virtual clock, click on **Leave the Floor** and then on **Restart the Program**.

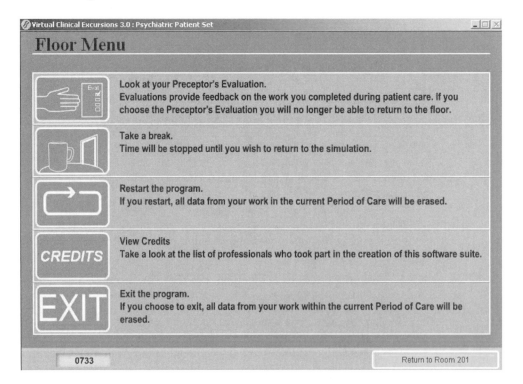

■ HOW TO PREPARE MEDICATIONS

From the Nurses' Station or the patient's room, you can access the Medication Room by clicking on the icon in the tool bar at the bottom of your screen to the left of the patient room numbers.

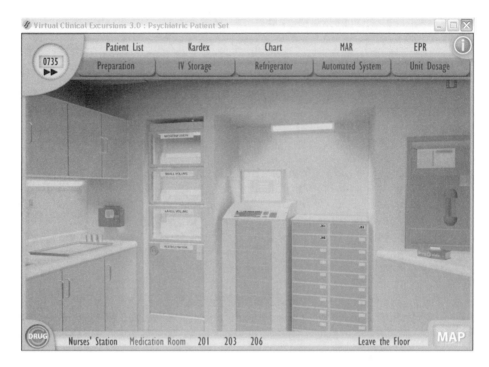

In the Medication Room you have access to the following (from left to right):

- A preparation area is located on the counter under the cabinets. To begin the medication preparation process, click on the tray on the counter or click on the **Preparation** icon at the top of the screen. The next screen leads you through a specific sequence (called the Preparation Wizard) to prepare medications one at a time for administration to a patient. However, no medication has been selected at this time. We will do this while working with a patient in *A Detailed Tour*. To exit this screen, click on **View Medication Room**.

- To the right of the cabinets (and above the refrigerator), IV storage bins are provided. Click on the bins themselves or on the **IV Storage** icon at the top of the screen. The bins are labeled **Microinfusion**, **Small Volume**, and **Large Volume**. Click on an individual bin to see a list of its contents. If you needed to prepare an IV medication at this time, you could click on the medication and its label would appear to the right under the patient's name. (*Note:* You can **Open** and **Close** any medication label by clicking the appropriate icon.) Next, you would click **Put Medication on Tray**. If you ever change your mind or decide that you have put the incorrect medication on the tray, you can reverse your actions by highlighting the medication on the tray and then clicking **Put Medication in Bin**. Click **Close Bin** in the right bottom corner to exit. **View Medication Room** brings you back to a full view of the entire room.

- A refrigerator is located under the IV storage bins to hold any medications that must be stored below room temperature. Click on the refrigerator door or on the **Refrigerator** icon at the top of the screen. Then click on the close-up view of the door to access the medications. When you are finished, click **Close Door** and then **View Medication Room**.

- To prepare controlled substances, click the **Automated System** icon at the top of the screen or click the computer monitor located to the right of the IV storage bins. A login screen will appear; your name and password are automatically filled in. Click **Login**. Select the patient for whom you wish to access medications; then select the correct medication drawer to open (they are stored alphabetically). Click **Open Drawer**, highlight the proper medication, and choose **Put Medication on Tray**. When you are finished, click **Close Drawer** and then **View Medication Room**.

- Next to the Automated System is a set of drawers identified by patient room number. To access these, click on the drawers or on the **Unit Dosage** icon at the top of the screen. This provides a close-up view of the drawers. To open a drawer, click on the room number of the patient you are working with. Next, click on the medication you would like to prepare for the patient, and a label will appear, listing the medication strength, units, and dosage per unit. To exit, click **Close Drawer**; then click **View Medication Room**.

At any time, you can learn about a medication you wish to prepare for a patient by clicking on the **Drug** icon in the bottom left corner of the medication room screen or by clicking the **Drug Guide** book on the counter to the right of the unit dosage drawers. The **Drug Guide** provides information about the medications commonly included in nursing drug handbooks. Nutritional supplements and maintenance intravenous fluid preparations are not included. Highlight a medication in the alphabetical list; relevant information about the drug will appear in the screen below. To exit, click **Return to Medication Room**.

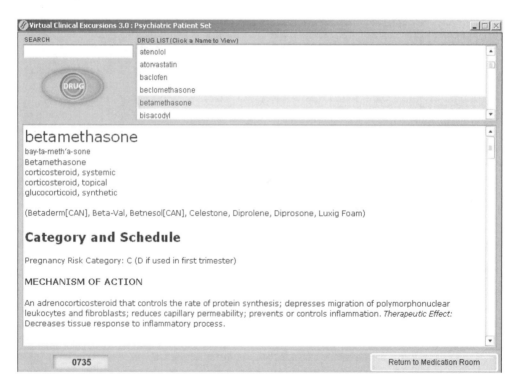

To access the MAR to review the medications ordered for a patient, click on the **MAR** icon located in the tool bar at the top of your screen and then click on the correct tab for your patient's room number. You may also click the **Review MAR** icon in the tool bar at the bottom of your screen from inside each medication storage area.

After you have chosen and prepared medications, go to the patient's room to administer them by clicking on the room number in the bottom tool bar. Inside the patient's room, click **Patient Care** and then **Medication Administration** and follow the proper administration sequence.

■ **PRECEPTOR'S EVALUATIONS**

When you have finished a session, click on **Leave the Floor** to go to the Floor Menu. At this point, you can click on the top icon (**Look at Your Preceptor's Evaluation**) to receive a score-card that provides feedback on the work you completed during patient care.

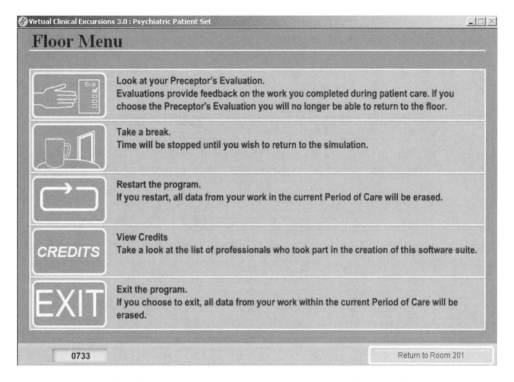

Evaluations are available for each patient you selected when you signed in for the current period of care. Click on the **Medication Scorecard** icon to see an example.

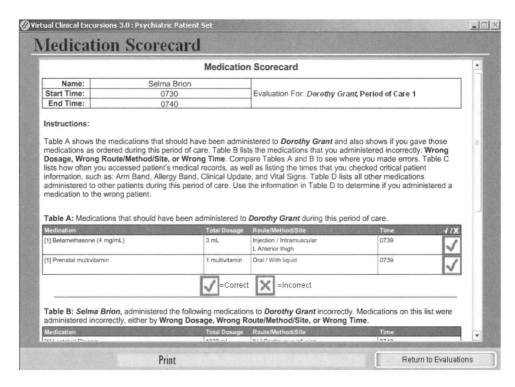

The scorecard compares the medications you administered to a patient during a period of care with what should have been administered. Table A lists the correct medications. Table B lists any medications that were administered incorrectly.

Remember, not every medication listed on the MAR should necessarily be given. For example, a patient might have an allergy to a drug that was ordered, or a medication might have been improperly transcribed to the MAR. Predetermined medication "errors" embedded within the program challenge you to exercise critical thinking skills and professional judgment when deciding to administer a medication, just as you would in a real hospital. Use all your available resources, such as the patient's chart and the MAR, to make your decision.

Table C lists the resources that were available to assist you in medication administration. It also documents whether and when you accessed these resources. For example, did you check the patient armband or perform a check of vital signs? If so, when?

You can click **Print** to get a copy of this report if needed. When you have finished reviewing the scorecard, click **Return to Evaluations** and then **Return to Menu**.

■ FLOOR MAP

To get a general sense of your location within the hospital, you can click on the **Map** icon found in the lower right corner of most of the screens in the *Virtual Clinical Excursions—Psychiatric* program. (*Note:* If you are following this quick tour step by step, you will need to **Restart the Program** from the Floor Menu, sign in again, and go to the Nurses' Station to access the map.) When you click the **Map** icon, a floor map appears, showing the layout of the floor you are currently on, as well as a directory of the patients and services on that floor. As you move your cursor over the directory list, the location of each room is highlighted on the map (and vice versa). The floor map can be accessed from the Nurses' Station, Medication Room, and each patient's room.

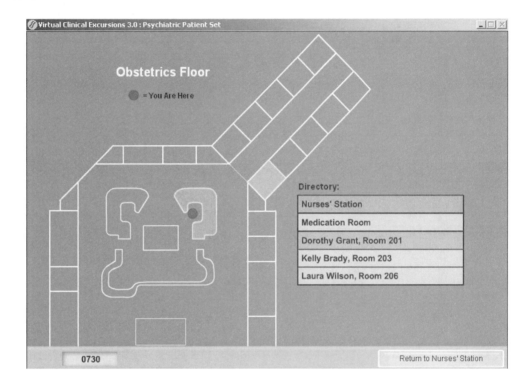

A DETAILED TOUR

If you wish to more thoroughly understand the capabilities of *Virtual Clinical Excursions—Psychiatric*, take a detailed tour by completing the following section. During this tour, we will work with a specific patient to introduce you to all the different components and learning opportunities available within the software.

■ WORKING WITH A PATIENT

Sign in and select the Obstetrics Floor for Period of Care 1 (0730-0815). From the Patient List, select Dorothy Grant in Room 201; however, do not go to the Nurses' Station yet.

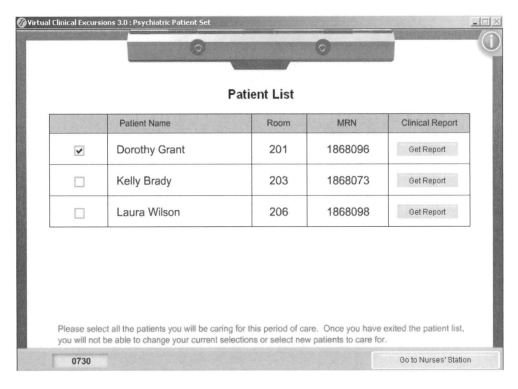

■ REPORT

In hospitals, when one shift ends and another begins, the outgoing nurse who attended a patient will give a verbal and sometimes a written summary of that patient's condition to the incoming nurse who will assume care for the patient. This summary is called a report and is an important source of data to provide an overview of a patient. Your first task is to get the clinical report on Dorothy Grant. To do this, click **Get Report** in the far right column in this patient's row. From a brief review of this summary, identify the problems and areas of concern that you will need to address for this patient.

When you have finished noting any areas of concern, click on **Go to Nurses' Station**.

■ CHARTS

You can access Dorothy Grant's chart from the Nurses' Station or from the patient's room (201).
From the Nurses' Station, click on the chart rack or on the **Chart** icon in the tool bar at the top
of your screen. Next, click on the chart labeled **201** to open the medical record for Dorothy
Grant. Click on the **Emergency Department** tab to view a record of why this patient was
admitted.

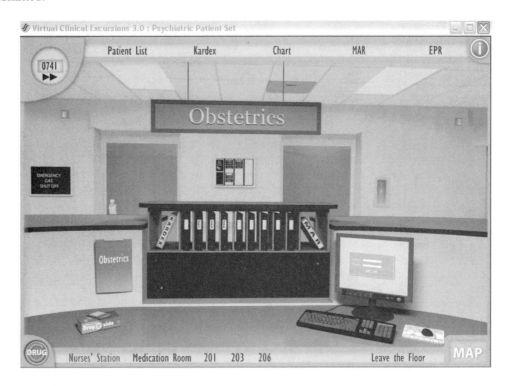

How many days has Dorothy Grant been in the hospital?

What tests were done upon her arrival in the Emergency Department and why?

What was her reason for admission?

You should also click on **Surgical Reports** to learn what procedures were performed and when.
Finally, review the **Nursing Admission** and **History and Physical** to learn about the health
history of this patient. When you are done reviewing the chart, click **Return to Nurses' Station**.

■ **MEDICATIONS**

Open the Medication Administration Record (MAR) by clicking on the **MAR** icon in the tool bar at the top of your screen. *Remember:* The MAR automatically opens to the first occupied room number on the floor—which is not necessarily your patient's room number! Since you need to access Dorothy Grant's MAR, click on tab **201** (her room number). Always make sure you are giving the *Right Drug to the Right Patient!*

Examine the list of medications ordered for Dorothy Grant. In the table below, list the medications that need to be given during this period of care (0730-0815). For each medication, note the dosage, route, and time to be given.

Time	Medication	Dosage	Route

Click on **Return to Nurses' Station**. Next, click on **201** on the bottom tool bar and then verify that you are indeed in Dorothy Grant's room. Select **Clinical Alerts** (the icon to the right of Initial Observations) to check for any emerging data that might affect your medication administration priorities. Next, go to the patient's chart (click on the **Chart** icon; then click on **201**). When the chart opens, select the **Physician's Orders** tab.

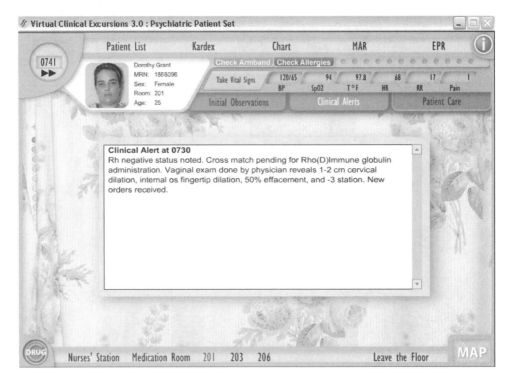

Review the orders. Have any new medications been ordered? Return to the MAR (click **Return to Room 201**; then click **MAR**). Verify that the new medications have been correctly transcribed to the MAR. Mistakes are sometimes made in the transcription process in the hospital setting, and it is sound practice to double-check any new order.

Are there any patient assessments you will need to perform before administering these medications? If so, return to Room 201 and click on **Patient Care** and then **Physical Assessment** to complete those assessments before proceeding.

Now click on the **Medication Room** icon in the tool bar at the bottom of your screen to locate and prepare the medications for Dorothy Grant.

In the Medication Room, you must access the medications for Dorothy Grant from the specific dispensing system in which each medication is stored. Locate each medication that needs to be given in this time period and click on **Put Medication on Tray** as appropriate. (*Hint:* Look in **Unit Dosage** drawer first.) When you are finished, click on **Close Drawer** and then on **View Medication Room**. Now click on the medication tray on the counter on the left side of the medication room screen to begin preparing the medications you have selected. (*Remember:* You can also click **Preparation** in the tool bar at the top of the screen.)

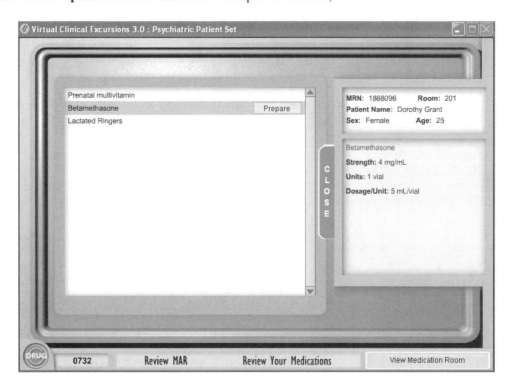

In the preparation area, you should see a list of the medications you put on the tray in the previous steps. Click on the first medication and then click **Prepare**. Follow the onscreen instructions of the Preparation Wizard, providing any data requested. As an example, let's follow the preparation process for betamethasone, one of the medications due to be administered to Dorothy Grant during this period of care. To begin, click to select **Betamethasone**; then click **Prepare**. Now work through the Preparation Wizard sequence as detailed below:

> Amount of medication in the ampule: Betamethasone 5 mL.
> Enter the amount of medication you will draw up into a syringe: **3 mL**.
> Click **Next**.
> Select the patient to receive the medication: **Room 201, Dorothy Grant**.
> Click **Finish**.
> Click **Return to Medication Room**.

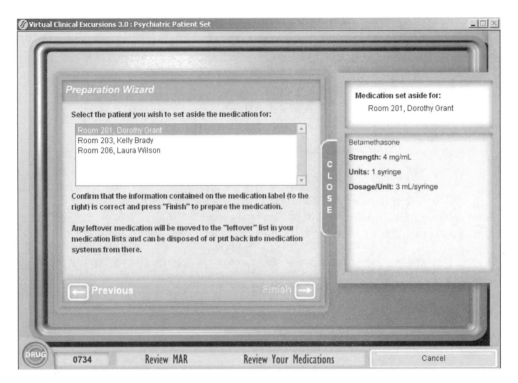

Follow this same basic process for the other medications due to be administered to Dorothy Grant during this period of care. (*Hint:* Look in **IV Storage** and **Automated System**.)

PREPARATION WIZARD EXCEPTIONS

- Some medications in *Virtual Clinical Excursions—Psychiatric* are prepared by the pharmacy (e.g., IV antibiotics) and taken to the patient room as a whole. This is common practice in most hospitals.
- Blood products are not administered by students through the *Virtual Clinical Excursions—Psychiatric* simulations since blood administration follows specific protocols not covered in this program.
- The *Virtual Clinical Excursions—Psychiatric* simulations do not allow for mixing more than one type of medication, such as regular and Lente insulins, in the same syringe. In the clinical setting, when multiple types of insulin are ordered for a patient, the regular insulin is drawn up first, followed by the longer-acting insulin. Insulin is always administered in a special unit-marked syringe.

Now return to Room 201 (click on **201** on the bottom tool bar) to administer Dorothy Grant's medications.

At any time during the medication administration process, you can perform a further review of systems, take vital signs, check information contained within the chart, or verify patient identity and allergies. Inside Dorothy Grant's room, click **Take Vital Signs**. (*Note:* These findings change over time to reflect the temporal changes you would find in a patient similar to Dorothy Grant.)

When you have gathered all the data you need, click on **Patient Care** and then select **Medica-tion Administration**. Any medications you prepared in the previous steps should be listed on the left side of your screen. Let's continue the administration process with the betamethasone ordered for Dorothy Grant. Click to highlight **Betamethasone** in the list of medications. Next, click on the down arrow to the right of **Select** and choose **Administer** from the drop-down menu. This will activate the Administration Wizard. Complete the Wizard sequence as follows:

- Route: **Injection**
- Method: **Intramuscular**
- Site: **Any** (choose one)
- Click **Administer to Patient** arrow.
- Would you like to document this administration in the MAR? **Yes**
- Click **Finish** arrow.

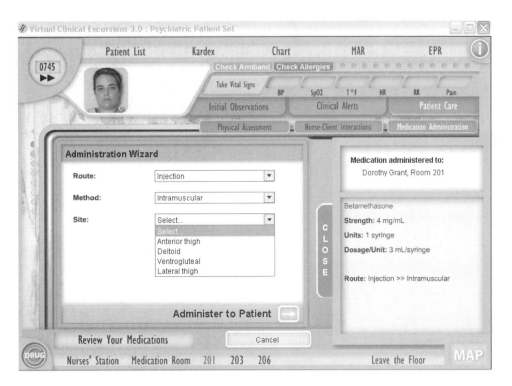

Your selections are recorded by a tracking system and evaluated on a Medication Scorecard stored under Preceptor's Evaluations. This scorecard can be viewed, printed, and given to your instructor. To access the Preceptor's Evaluations, click on **Leave the Floor**. When the Floor Menu appears, select **Look at Your Preceptor's Evaluation**. Then click on **Medication Scorecard** inside the box with Dorothy Grant's name (see example on the following page).

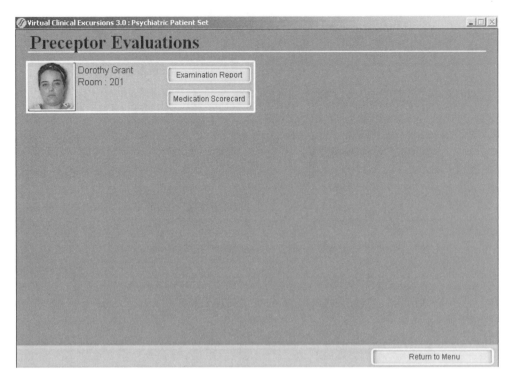

■ MEDICATION SCORECARD

- First, review Table A. Was betamethasone given correctly? Did you give the other medications as ordered?
- Table B shows you which (if any) medications you gave incorrectly.
- Table C addresses the resources used for Dorothy Grant. Did you access the patient's chart, MAR, EPR, or Kardex as needed to make safe medication administration decisions?
- Did you check the patient's armband to verify her identity? Did you check whether your patient had any known allergies to medications? Were vital signs taken?

When you have finished reviewing the scorecard, click **Return to Evaluations** and then **Return to Menu**.

■ VITAL SIGNS

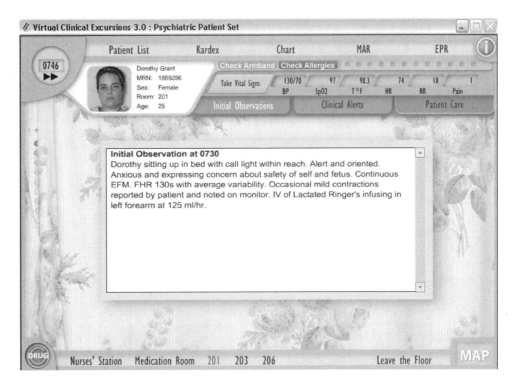

Vital signs, often considered the traditional "signs of life," include body temperature, heart rate, respiratory rate, blood pressure, oxygen saturation of the blood, and pain level.

Inside Dorothy Grant's room, click **Take Vital Signs**. (*Note:* If you are following this detailed tour step by step, you will need to **Restart the Program** from the Floor Menu, sign in again, and navigate to Room 201.) Collect vital signs for this patient and record them below. Note the time at which you collected each of these data. (*Remember:* You can take vital signs at any time. The data change over time to reflect the temporal changes you would find in a patient similar to Dorothy Grant.)

Vital Signs	Findings/Time
Blood pressure	
O₂ saturation	
Heart rate	
Respiratory rate	
Temperature	
Pain rating	

After you are done, click on the **EPR** icon located in the tool bar at the top of the screen. Your username and password are automatically provided. Click on **Login** to enter the EPR. To access Dorothy Grant's records, click on the down arrow next to Patient and choose her room number, **201**. Select **Vital Signs** as the category. Next, in the empty time column on the far right, record the vital signs data you just collected in Dorothy Grant's room. (*Note:* If you need help with this process, see page 16.) Now compare these findings with the data you collected earlier for this patient's vital signs. Use these earlier findings to establish a baseline for each of the vital signs.

    a.   Are any of the data you collected significantly different from the baseline for a particular vital sign?

        Circle One: Yes   No

    b.   If "Yes," which data are different?

■ PHYSICAL ASSESSMENT

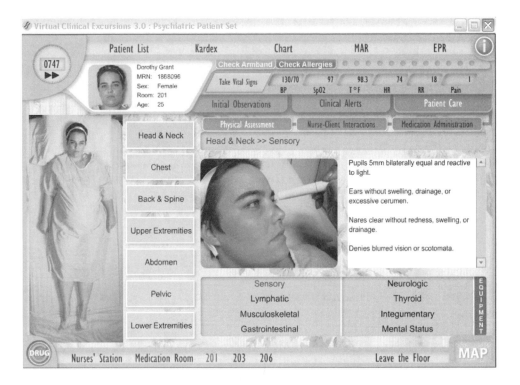

After you have finished examining the EPR for vital signs, click **Exit EPR** to return to Room 201. Click **Patient Care** and then **Physical Assessment**. Think about the information you received in the report at the beginning of this shift, as well as what you may have learned about this patient from the chart. Based on this, what area(s) of examination should you pay most attention to at this time? Is there any equipment you should be monitoring? Conduct a physical assessment of the body areas and systems that you consider priorities for Dorothy Grant. For example, select **Head & Neck**; then click on and assess **Sensory** and **Lymphatic**. Complete any other assessment(s) you think are necessary at this time. In the following table, record the data you collected during this examination.

Area of Examination	Findings
Head & Neck Sensory	
Head & Neck Lymphatic	

After you have finished collecting these data, return to the EPR. Compare the data that were already in the record with those you just collected.

a. Are any of the data you collected significantly different from the baselines for this patient?

Circle One: Yes   No

b. If "Yes," which data are different?

■ **NURSE-CLIENT INTERACTIONS**

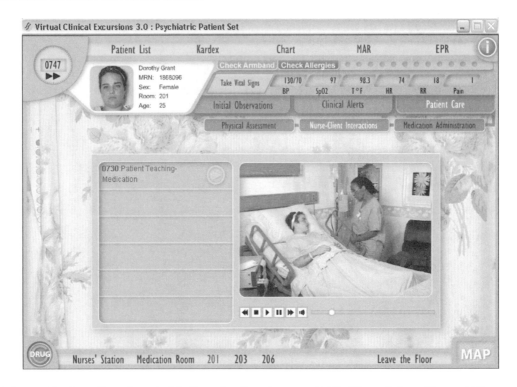

Click on **Patient Care** from inside Dorothy Grant's room (201). Now click on **Nurse-Client Interactions** to access a short video titled **Patient Teaching—Medication**, which is available for viewing at or after 0730 (based on the virtual clock in the upper left corner of your screen; see *Note* below). To begin the video, click on the white arrow next to its title. You will observe a nurse communicating with Dorothy Grant. There are many variations of nursing practice, some exemplifying "best" practice and some not. Note whether the nurse in this interaction displays professional behavior and compassionate care. Are her words congruent with what is going on with the patient? Does this interaction "feel right" to you? If not, how would you handle this situation differently? Explain.

Note: If the video you wish to view is not listed, this means you have not yet reached the correct virtual time to view that video. Check the virtual clock; you may return to access the video once its designated time has occurred—as long as you do so within the same period of care. Or you can click on the fast-forward icon within the virtual clock to advance the time by 2-minute intervals. You will then need to click again on **Patient Care** and **Nurse-Client Interactions** to refresh the screen.

At least one Nurse-Client Interactions video is available during each period of care. Viewing these videos can help you learn more about what is occurring with a patient at a certain time and also prompt you to discern between nurse communications that are ideal and those that need improvement. Compassionate care and the ability to communicate clearly are essential components of delivering quality nursing care, and it is during your clinical time that you will begin to refine these skills.

■ COLLECTING AND EVALUATING DATA

Each of the activities you perform in the Patient Care environment generates a significant amount of assessment data. Remember that after you collect data, you can record your findings in the EPR. You can also review the EPR, patient's chart, videos, and MAR at any time. You will get plenty of practice collecting and then evaluating data in context of the patient's course.

Now, here's an important question for you:

> Did the previous sequence of exercises provide the most efficient way to assess Dorothy Grant?

For example, you went to the patient's room to get vital signs, then back to the EPR to enter data and compare your findings with extant data. Next, you went back to the patient's room to do a physical examination, then again back to the EPR to enter and review data. If this back-and-forth process of data collection and recording seemed inefficient, remember the following:

- Plan all of your nursing activities to maximize efficiency, while at the same time optimizing the quality of patient care. (Think about what data you might need before performing certain tasks. For example, do you need to check a heart rate before administering a cardiac medication or check an IV site before starting an infusion?)

- You collect a tremendous amount of data when you work with a patient. Very few people can accurately remember all these data for more than a few minutes. Develop efficient assessment skills, and record data as soon as possible after collecting them.

- Assessment data are only the starting point for the nursing process.

Make a clear distinction between these first exercises and how you actually provide nursing care. These initial exercises were designed to involve you actively in the use of different software components. This workbook focuses on sensible practices for implementing the nursing process in ways that ensure the highest-quality care of patients.

Most important, remember that a human being changes through time, and that these changes include both the physical and psychosocial facets of a person as a living organism. Think about this for a moment. Some patients may change physically in a very short time (a patient with emerging myocardial infarction) or more slowly (a patient with a chronic illness). Patients' overall physical and psychosocial conditions may improve or deteriorate. They may have effective coping skills and familial support, or they may feel alone and full of despair. In fact, each individual is a complex mix of physical and psychosocial elements, and at least some of these elements usually change through time.

Thus it is crucial that you *DO NOT* think of the nursing process as a simple one-time, five-step procedure consisting of assessment, nursing diagnosis, planning, implementation, and evaluation. Rather, the nursing process should be utilized as a creative and systematic approach to delivering nursing care. Furthermore, because all living organisms are constantly changing, we must apply the nursing process over and over. Each time we follow the nursing process for an individual patient, we refine our understanding of that patient's physical and psychosocial conditions based on collection and analysis of many different types of data. *Virtual Clinical Excursions—Psychiatric* will help you develop both the creativity and the systematic approach needed to become a nurse who is equipped to deliver the highest-quality care to all patients.

REDUCING MEDICATION ERRORS

Earlier in this detailed tour, you learned the basic steps of medication preparation and administration. The following simulations will allow you to practice those skills further—with an increased emphasis on reducing medication errors by using the Medication Scorecard to evaluate your work.

Sign in to work on the Obstetrics Floor at Pacific View Regional Hospital for Period of Care 1. (*Note:* If you are already working with another patient or during another period of care, click on **Leave the Floor** and then **Restart the Program**; then sign in.)

From the Patient List, select Dorothy Grant. Then click on **Go to Nurses' Station**. Complete the following steps to prepare and administer medications to Dorothy Grant.

- Click on **Medication Room**.
- Click on **MAR** and then on tab **201** to determine prn medications that have been ordered for Dorothy Grant. (*Note:* You may click on **Review MAR** at any time to verify the correct medication orders. Always remember to check the patient name on the MAR to make sure you have the correct patient's record—you must click on the correct room number tab within the MAR.) Click on **Return to Medication Room** after reviewing the correct MAR.
- Click on **Unit Dosage** (or on the Unit Dosage cabinet); from the close-up view, click on drawer **201**.
- Select the medications you would like to administer. After each selection, click **Put Medication on Tray**. When you are finished selecting medications, click **Close Drawer** and then **View Medication Room**.
- Click on **Automated System** (or on the Automated System unit itself). Click **Login**.
- On the next screen, specify the correct patient and drawer location.
- Select the medication you would like to administer and click **Put Medication on Tray**. Repeat this process if you wish to administer other medications from the Automated System.
- When you are finished, click **Close Drawer** and **View Medication Room**.
- From the Medication Room, click **Preparation** (or on the preparation tray).
- From the list of medications on your tray, highlight the correct medication to administer and click **Prepare**.
- This activates the Preparation Wizard. Supply any requested information; then click **Next**.
- Now select the correct patient to receive this medication and click **Finish**.
- Repeat the previous three steps until all medications that you want to administer are prepared.
- You can click **Review Your Medications** and then **Return to Medication Room** when ready. Once you are back in the Medication Room, go directly to Dorothy Grant's room by clicking on **201** at the bottom of the screen.
- Inside the patient's room, administer the medication, utilizing the six rights of medication administration. After you have collected the appropriate assessment data and are ready for administration, click **Patient Care** and then **Medication Administration**. Verify that the correct patient and medication(s) appear in the left-hand window. Highlight the first medication you wish to administer; then click the down arrow next to Select. From the drop-down menu, select **Administer** and complete the Administration Wizard by providing any information requested. When the Wizard stops asking for information, click **Administer to Patient**. Specify **Yes** when asked whether this administration should be recorded in the MAR. Finally, click **Finish**.

■ **SELF-EVALUATION**

Now let's see how you did during your medication administration!

• Click on **Leave the Floor** at the bottom of your screen. From the Floor Menu, select **Look at Your Preceptor's Evaluation**. Then click on **Medication Scorecard**.

The following exercises will help you identify medication errors, investigate possible reasons for these errors, and reduce or prevent medication errors in the future.

1. Start by examining Table A. These are the medications you should have given to Dorothy Grant during this period of care. If each of the medications in Table A has a ✓ by it, then you made no errors. Congratulations!

If any medication has an X by it, then you made one or more medication errors.

Compare Tables A and B to determine which of the following types of errors you made: Wrong Dose, Wrong Route/Method/Site, or Wrong Time. Follow these steps:
   a. Find medications in Table A that were given incorrectly.
   b. Now see if those same medications are in Table B, which shows what you actually administered to Dorothy Grant.
   c. Comparing Tables A and B, match the Strength, Dose, Route/Method/Site, and Time for each medication you administered incorrectly.
   d. Then, using the form below, list the medications given incorrectly and mark the errors you made for each medication.

Medication	Strength	Dosage	Route	Method	Site	Time
	❑	❑	❑	❑	❑	❑
	❑	❑	❑	❑	❑	❑
	❑	❑	❑	❑	❑	❑
	❑	❑	❑	❑	❑	❑

2. To help you reduce future medication errors, consider the following list of possible reasons for errors.

   • Did not check drug against MAR for correct patient, correct date, correct time, correct drug, and correct dose.
   • Did not check drug dose against MAR three times.
   • Did not open the unit dose package in the patient's room.
   • Did not correctly identify the patient using two identifiers.
   • Did not administer the drug on time.
   • Did not verify patient allergies.
   • Did not check the patient's current condition or vital sign parameters.
   • Did not consider why the patient would be receiving this drug.
   • Did not question why the drug was in the patient's drawer.
   • Did not check the physician's order and/or check with the pharmacist when there was a question about the drug or dose.
   • Did not verify that no adverse effects had occurred from a previous dose.

Based on the list of possibilities you just reviewed, determine how you made each error and record the reason in the form below:

Medication	Reason for Error

3. Look again at Table B. Are there medications listed that are not in Table A? If so, you gave a medication to Dorothy Grant that she should not have received. Complete the following exercises to help you understand how such an error might have been made.

   a. Perhaps you gave a medication that was on Dorothy Grant's MAR for this period of care, without recognizing that a change had occurred in the patient's condition, which should have caused you to reconsider. Review patient records as necessary and complete the following form:

Medication	Possible Reasons Not to Give This Medication

   b. Another possibility is that you gave Dorothy Grant a medication that should have been given at a different time. Check her MAR and complete the form below to determine whether you made a Wrong Time error:

Medication	Given to Dorothy Grant at What Time	Should Have Been Given at What Time

c. Maybe you gave another patient's medication to Dorothy Grant. In this case, you made a Wrong Patient error. Check the MARs of other patients and use the form below to determine whether you made this type of error:

Medication	Given to Dorothy Grant	Should Have Been Given to

4. The Medication Scorecard provides some other interesting sources of information. For example, if there is a medication selected for Dorothy Grant but it was not given to her, there will be an X by that medication in Table A, but it will not appear in Table B. In that case, you might have given this medication to some other patient, which is another type of Wrong Patient error. To investigate further, look at Table D, which lists the medications you gave to other patients. See whether you can find any medications ordered for Dorothy Grant that were given to another patient by mistake. However, before you make any decisions, be sure to cross-check the MAR for other patients because the same medication may have been ordered for multiple patients. Use the following form to record your findings:

Medication	Should Have Been Given to Dorothy Grant	Given by Mistake to

5. Now take some time to review the medication exercises you just completed. Use the form below to create an overall analysis of what you have learned. Once again, record each of the medication errors you made, including the type of each error. Then, for each error you made, indicate specifically what you would do differently to prevent this type of error from occurring again.

Medication	Type of Error	Error Prevention Tactic

Submit this form to your instructor if required as a graded assignment, or simply use these exercises to improve your understanding of medication errors and how to reduce them.

Name: _____   Date: _____

The following icons are used throughout this workbook to help you quickly identify particular activities and assignments:

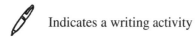 Indicates a reading assignment—tells you which textbook chapter(s) you should read before starting each lesson

Indicates a writing activity

Marks the beginning of an interactive CD-ROM activity—signals you to open or return to your *Virtual Clinical Excursions—Psychiatric* CD-ROM

Indicates additional CD-ROM instructions

Indicates questions and activities that require you to consult your textbook

Indicates the approximate time required to complete an exercise

LESSON **1**

Mental Health and Mental Illness

/O&O **Reading Assignment:** Mental Health and Mental Illness (Chapter 1)

Patient: Harry George, Medical-Surgical Floor, Room 401

Goal: To understand the role of the nurse in caring for a patient along the mental health and illness continuum.

Objectives:

- Define mental health.
- Discuss the concepts of the mental health and mental illness continuum.
- Identify mental illness prevalence rates in the United States.
- Understand the 5 axes of the DSM-IV-TR.
- Understand the relationship between the DSM-IV-TR and NANDA.
- Understand the role of the nurse in caring for a patient along the mental health and mental illness continuum.
- Define evidence-based nursing practice.

In this lesson you will learn about the the role of the nurse in caring for the patient along the continuum of care from mental health to mental illness.

Exercise 1

Clinical Preparation: Writing Activity

30 minutes

1. Mental health is defined as the

   a. ability to think clearly and rationally, solve problems, and use good judgment.
   b. ability to engage in productive activities, such as work.
   c. ability to relate to others and have close, loving relationships.
   d. ability to cope with typical stresses of life.
   (e.) all of the above.

2. Below, place an X next to each statement that is true regarding the concepts of mental health and mental illness.

   _X_ Many forms of unusual behavior may be tolerated, depending on the cultural norms.

   _X_ Mentally ill individuals are those who violate social norms.

   _X_ There are many influences that impact the mental health of an individual, such as heredity, culture, health practices, support, and life stressors.

   ____ Mental illness is defined as being different or strange.

   _X_ Mental health means one is logical and rational.

   _X_ All human behavior lies somewhere along a continuum of mental health and illness.

3. Discuss resilience as it relates to mental health.

   Resilience is closely associated with the process of adapting and helps people facing tragedies, loss, trauma, and severe stress. It also means that rather than falling victim to negative emotions, resilient people recognize the feeling, readily deal with them, and learn from the experience.

4. Four of the ten leading causes of disability in the United States are caused by

   OCD, major depression, schizophrenia, bipolar disorder

5. The National Institute of Mental Health publishes prevalence rates of mental illness in the United States. Which of the following statement(s) is/are true?

   a. One in five adults has a diagnosable mental disorder.
   b. Substance-related disorders are not a category in the DSM-IV-TR.
   c. 14.8 million people in the United States have major depressive disorder.
   d. Posttraumatic stress disorder occurs only after involvement in military conflict.
   (e.) Both a and c are true.

6. The Diagnostic and Statistical Manual of Mental Disorders (DSM-IV-TR) requires judgments to be made on five axes, requiring the practitioner to consider a broad range of information. Match each specific axis to its description.

Axis		**Description**
_B_	Axis I	a. Psychosocial and environmental problems that may affect the diagnosis, treatment, and prognosis of a mental disorder
_D_	Axis II	
_E_	Axis III	b. Collection of signs and symptoms that together establish a specific disorder
_A_	Axis IV	c. An assessment of psychological, social, and occupational functioning during the past year (GAF)
_C_	Axis V	d. Personality disorders and mental retardation
		e. Medical conditions thought to be relevant to the mental disorder

7. Discuss the relationship between the Diagnostic and Statistical Manual (DSM-IV-TR) and the North American Nursing Diagnosis Association International (NANDA-I).

DSM IV TR is used to identify Medical diagnosis for clients with mental health disorders. NANDA is used for nursing diagnosis r/t the medical diagnosis that nurse can treat.

8. Define evidence-based practice.

It is a collection, interpretation and integration of valid, important, and applicable patient-reported, clinician observed, and researched derived evidence

Exercise 2

 CD-ROM Activity

30 minutes

- Sign in to work at Pacific View Regional Hospital on the Medical-Surgical Floor for Period of Care 1. (*Note:* If you are already in the virtual hospital from a previous exercise, click on **Leave the Floor** and then **Restart the Program** to get to the sign-in window.)
- From the Patient List, select Harry George (Room 401).
- Click on **Go to Nurses' Station**.
- Click on **Chart** and then on **401**.
- Read the **History and Physical**.
- Next, read the **Nursing Admission**.

1. What are the stressors that led up to Harry George's current life situation?

   a. Motorcycle accident
   b. Chronic left foot bone infection and severe pain
   c. Estrangement from wife and two sons
   d. Loss of job
   e. Homelessness
   f. All of the above

2. After reviewing the History and Physical and the Nursing Admission, list Harry George's medical diagnoses below. For each diagnosis, identify potential nursing problems associated with that diagnosis.

Medical Diagnoses	Nursing Problems
Cellulitis (L) foot c/ osteomylitis	Infection Pain
Type 2 diabetes	Nutrition Blood sugar
Alcoholism	Withdrawals

3. Match each type of health education intervention with the specific health topics Harry George will need during hospitalization and after discharge.

Type of Health Education Interventions

 Increase awareness of issues related to health and illness

 Increase understanding of potential stressors, possible outcomes, and alternative coping responses

 Increase knowledge of where and how to obtain resources

 Increase actual abilities

Specific Health Topic

a. Developing healthy coping skills, such as stress reduction; developing motivation and self-esteem; problem solving; and stress management

b. Learning how to become clean and sober, caring for self, managing pain and diabetes, and smoking cessation

c. Finding housing, finding/keeping job, and locating family members

d. Dealing with loss of family and job, homelessness, and pain

4. How important is pain management in Harry George's rehabilitation and recovery?

It is priority because patients don't function well with too much pain

5. In view of Harry George's current living situation and 4-year history of alcoholism, what do you think would be the best type of program to help him quit drinking upon discharge?

a. Community-based sober living house
b. Inpatient alcohol/drug treatment program
c. Outpatient visits with a drug/alcohol counselor
d. Does not really matter since he will not stop drinking

6. Below and on the next page, describe the challenges that Harry George faces in his recovery in the following areas.

Area of Rehabilitation/Recovery	Challenge
Activities of daily living (ADL)	— Pain
Interpersonal relationships	— Opening up to people — Coping
Self-esteem	
Motivation	
Illness management	

Area of Rehabilitation/Recovery	Challenge
Strengths	

7. What hospital-based resources does the nurse have available to help Harry George with the community needs he will have after discharge?

Smoker Cessation
Social Services
Nutritionist

8. Using information from your textbook and taking into consideration Harry George's history and current needs, discuss how a positive change in his living/social environment could affect his rehabilitation and recovery.

It would allow him to have a speedy recovery. and get his life on track

LESSON **2**

Culturally Relevant
Mental Health Nursing

Reading Assignment: Cultural Implications for Psychiatric Mental Health Nursing
(Chapter 6)
The Nursing Process and Standards of Care for Psychiatric
Mental Health Nursing (Chapter 8)

Patient: Carlos Reyes, Skilled Nursing Floor, Room 504

Goal: To be able to understand cultural aspects of psychiatric nursing care.

Objectives:

- Understand how culture helps define mental health and illness.
- Define culturally competent care.
- Define practice barriers to providing culturally competent care.
- Describe methods the nurse can use to overcome barriers to culturally competent care.
- Describe methods the nurse can use to provide culturally competent care.
- Understand the role language and culture plays in the assessment, diagnosis, and treatment of mental illness.
- Examine the difference between a translator and an interpreter.

Exercise 1

Clinical Preparation: Writing Activity

15 minutes

1. Psychiatric mental health nurses must practice _culturally relevant ~~too~~_ nursing to meet the needs of culturally diverse patients.

2. Place an X next to each true statement regarding culture and mental health and illness.

   X   Each cultural group has cultural beliefs, values, and practices that guide its members in ways of thinking and acting.

   _____ The framework that describes mental health and illness in the United States is based on Eastern thought.

   _____ Culture defines the differences between mental health and illness.

   _____ Deviance from cultural expectations is considered to be a problem and is usually seen by the cultural group as an "illness."

   X   The same thoughts and behaviors that are considered mental health in one culture can be considered an illness in another culture.

3. In providing care to culturally diverse populations, the nurse will encounter barriers in practice and must be knowledgeable about methods to overcome these barriers. Listed below and on the next page are three practice issues and their associated barriers. Complete the table by listing ways the nurse can overcome each barrier.

Practice Issue	Barrier	Methods to Overcome Barrier
Communication	Limited proficiency in language, meaning of nonverbal communication	Get an interpreter Cultural broker

Practice Issue	Barrier	Methods to Overcome Barrier
Diagnosis	Misdiagnosis; use of culturally inappropriate psychometric diagnostic tools	*Use the DSM-IV-TR for diagnosing mental illness*
Pharmacodynamics	Genetic variations in drug metabolism found in people of all ethnicities	*- Keep abreast of current findings related to the drugs* *- Carry out cultural assessments c/ all patients* *- Carefully monitor and document drug responses and give lowest possible safe dose* *- Incorporate cultural context in nursing education*

4. Culturally competent care is defined as attitudes and behaviors that enable a nurse to work effectively within a patient's cultural context. Therefore nurses need to adjust their

   _practices_____ to meet their patients' cultural beliefs and practices, needs, and preferences.

5. Using the process of Cultural Competence in delivering mental health care, describe how the psychiatric mental health nurse can develop culturally competent care in the following areas.

Area	Nurse's Behavior
Cultural awareness	
Cultural knowledge	
Cultural encounters	
Cultural skill	
Cultural desire	

6. In order to perform a cultural assessment on Carlos Reyes, there are key questions that are important to include. Place an X next to each question you think would be important to include in the assessment.

_____   How old are you?

_X_   What is your primary language? Would you like a translator?

_____   How would you describe your cultural background?

_____   Who do you live with? Who are you close to?

_X_   Are there special foods you like to eat?

_____   How is your illness viewed by your culture?

_____   How tall are you? How much do you weigh?

_X_   What do you do to get better when you are medically ill? Mentally ill?

7. For patients who do not speak English or who have difficulties with the language, federal law mandates the use of a trained translator. List the skills of a professionally trained translator, and explain how they are different from those of an interpreter.

Exercise 2

  CD-ROM Activity

45 minutes

- Sign in to work at Pacific View Regional Hospital on the Skilled Nursing Floor for Period of Care 1. (*Note:* If you are already in the virtual hospital from a previous exercise, click on **Leave the Floor** and then **Restart the Program** to get to the sign-in window.)
- From the Patient List, select Carlos Reyes (Room 504).
- Click on **Go to Nurses' Station**.
- Click on **Chart** and then on **504**.
- Read the **History and Physical** and **Nursing Admission** records.

1. According to the medical record, Carlos Reyes' cultural background is

   Hispanic.

2. What are some characteristics of the culture you identified in question 1?

   Hispanic
   Catholic

3. Discuss the cultural factors present in caring for Carlos Reyes.

   - Daughter describes father as a loyal and devoted husband and father
   - Is Catholic -- does not attend church
   - SHe would like last rites if father were to die
   - Daughter would like a Catholic priest (only)

→ • Click on **Return to Nurses' Station**.
   • Click on **504** at the bottom of the screen.
   • Click on **Patient Care** and then on **Nurse-Client Interactions**.
   • To answer questions 4-8, you will need to select and view the video titles listed below. (*Note:* Check the virtual clock to see whether enough time has elapsed. You can use the fast-forward feature to advance the time by 2-minute intervals if the video is not yet available. Then click on **Patient Care** and **Nurse-Client Interactions** to refresh the screen.)
     • 0740: Family Teaching—Medication
     • 0745: Drowsiness—Contributing Factor
     • 0750: Assessment—Level of Assistance
   • After viewing the above three videos, click on the **Drug** icon in the lower left corner of your screen. Use the Search box or the scroll bar to find information on oxazepam.

4. The two interventions the nurse used to answer the concerns of Carlos Reyes' son regarding

   his father's drowsiness were <u>family teaching</u> and

   <u>Side effects of</u> the patient's medications as a cause for drowsiness.

5. What other actions could the nurse have taken?

   — She should have explained exactly what would happen if they removed the drug abruptly.
   — Print out med information

6. Explain the indication for oxazepam and the effect it has on brain function. Identify the side effect that was concerning Carlos Reyes' son.

Indications
—Management of anxiety, anxiety associate c/ depression

CNS Side effects
—dizziness
—drowsiness
—confusion
—hang over
—head over
—impaired memory

—mental depression
—paradoxical excitation
—slurred speech

7. What aspects of the mental status exam is the nurse attempting to assess?

   a. Appearance, speech, motor activity, and interaction
   b. Level of consciousness
   c. Emotional state: mood and affect
   d. All of the above

8. What level of assistance will Carlos Reyes need in order to sit up and eat his breakfast? Discuss the role of his family at mealtime.

- Elevate the HOB
- 1 assisst
- Set up tray
- Teach family how to feed
- aspiration precautious

LESSON **3** _____

Therapeutic Relationships

_____

Reading Assignment: Therapeutic Relationships (Chapter 9)
Communication and the Clinical Interview (Chapter 10)

Patients: Jacquline Catanazaro, Medical-Surgical Floor, Room 402
Kathryn Doyle, Skilled Nursing Floor, Room 503

Goal: Demonstrate an understanding of the importance of the therapeutic nurse-patient relationship and be able to identify and use therapeutic communication techniques with patients.

Objectives:

- Understand the characteristics and goals of the therapeutic nurse-patient relationship.
- Identify the personal qualities of the nurse that are necessary to communicate effectively.
- Describe the qualities of genuineness, empathy, and positive regard in the therapeutic nurse-patient relationship.
- Discuss the verbal and nonverbal components of communication.
- Discuss types of boundary issues and their importance to the nurse-patient relationship.
- Identify transference and countertransference in the therapeutic nurse-patient relationship.
- Describe the phases of a therapeutic nurse-patient relationship.
- Observe and identify effective communication techniques used by the nurse in nurse-patient interactions.

Exercise 1

 Clinical Preparation: Writing Activity

30 minutes

1. The therapeutic nurse-patient relationship is the basis of all psychiatric nursing treatment approaches, regardless of the goal. List the characteristics and goals of the therapeutic relationship below.

Characteristics of a Therapeutic Relationship	Goals of a Therapeutic Relationship
- The needs of the patient are identified and explored	- Facilitate communication of distressing thoughts and feelings
• Clear boundaries are established	- Assisting pt's c/ problem solving to help c/ ADLs
• Alternate problem-solving approaches are taken	
- New coping skills may be developed	
- Behavioral change is encouraged	

2. Which personal behaviors, qualities, and skills must the nurse have in order to communicate therapeutically with patients? Select all that apply.

___X___ Accountability

___X___ Focus on the patient's needs

___X___ Clinical competence

___X___ Delaying judgment

_____ Self-awareness

_____ Understanding of one's own values and beliefs

3. Discuss communication and the importance of its verbal and nonverbal components.

Verbal communication consists of all the words a person speaks, whereas in nonverbal communication, there are nonverbal behaviors. These consists of the tone of voice, emphasis on certain words, and the manner in which a person paces speech. Other common examples of non verbal communication (often called cues) are physical appearance, facial expressions, body posture, amount of eye contact, eye cast, hand gestures, sighs, fidgeting, and yawning.

4. Describe the personal qualities of genuineness, empathy, and positive regard that a nurse must have in order to establish and maintain a therapeutic relationship.

Genuiness is the same as self-awareness of one's feelings as they arise within the relationship and the ability to communicate them when appropriate. Genuiness is when the person displays the same thing on the outside that is on the inside. It is conveyed by listening to and communicating c̄ patients without distorting their messages and being clear and concrete in communication. Empathy involves accurately perceiving the patient's situation, perspective, and feelings; communicating one's understanding to the patient and checking with the patient for accuracy; and acting on this understanding in a helpful (therapeutic) way toward the patient.

5. Establishing and maintaining boundaries in the nurse-patient relationship are challenging tasks. Boundaries are always at risk for being blurred. Two common circumstances that can produce blurring of boundaries are when the relationship slips into a social context and

when the nurse's need (for attention, affection, emotional support) are met at the expense of the patient's needs.

6. Role blurring is often the result of unrecognized transference or countertransference. Match each term with its definition.

Term	Definition
_a_ Countertransference	a. Unconscious response in which the patient experiences feelings and attitudes toward the nurse originally associated with other significant figures in the patient's life.
_b_ Transference	b. Response used by the nurse; the specific emotional response to the qualities of the patient. This is inappropriate to the content and context of the therapeutic relationship.

7. The three phases of the nurse-patient relationship are ___orientation___,

   ___Working___, and ___termination___.

8. Match the phase of the nurse-patient relationship with its characteristics.

   Phase

   _b_ Orientation

   _c_ Working

   _a_ Termination

   Characteristics

   a. Signifies a loss for both the patient and nurse; goals and objectives are summarized, and progress is reviewed; possible regression.

   b. Trust is established, relationship is defined, contracts are established, and confidentiality and termination are discussed.

   c. Focus is on maintenance, gathering more information, promoting patient's strengths, facilitating behavioral change, overcoming resistance, evaluating problems and goals, and promoting practice and expression of alternative adaptive behaviors.

Exercise 2

  CD-ROM Activity

🕐 30 minutes

- Sign in to work at Pacific View Regional Hospital on the Medical-Surgical Floor for Period of Care 1. (*Note:* If you are already in the virtual hospital from a previous exercise, click on **Leave the Floor** and then **Restart the Program** to get to the sign-in window.)
- From the Patient List, select Jacquline Catanazaro (Room 402).
- Click on **Go to Nurses' Station** and then on **402** at the bottom of the screen.
- Click on **Patient Care** and then on **Nurse-Client Interactions**.
- Select and view the video titled **0730: Intervention—Airway**. (*Note:* Check the virtual clock to see whether enough time has elapsed. You can use the fast-forward feature to advance the time by 2-minute intervals if the video is not yet available. Then click on **Patient Care** and **Nurse-Client Interactions** to refresh the screen.)

1. As you observe the 0730 video, make note of the therapeutic verbal and nonverbal communication techniques the nurse uses. Record these in the first column of the table below. Then, for each technique you identify, list specific examples of verbal and nonverbal communication used by the nurse that demonstrate the technique.

Therapeutic Communication Techniques Used by Nurse	Specific Examples of Nurse Communication
Verbal	
Nonverbal	

Now let's jump ahead in time to observe a later interaction between the nurse and this patient.

 • Click on **Leave the Floor** and then on **Restart the Program**.
- Sign in to work on the Medical-Surgical Floor for Period of Care 2.
- From the Patient List, select Jacquline Catanazaro (Room 402).
- Click on **Go to Nurses' Station** and then on **402** at the bottom of the screen.
- Click on **Patient Care** and then on **Nurse-Client Interactions**.
- Select and view the video titled **1115: Assessment—Readiness to Learn**. (*Note:* Check the virtual clock to see whether enough time has elapsed. You can use the fast-forward feature to advance the time by 2-minute intervals if the video is not yet available. Then click on **Patient Care** and **Nurse-Client Interactions** to refresh the screen.)

2. As you observe the 1115 video, make note of the therapeutic verbal and nonverbal communication techniques the nurse uses. Record these in the first column of the table below. Then, for each technique you identify, list specific examples of verbal and nonverbal communication used by the nurse that demonstrate the technique.

Therapeutic Communication Techniques Used by Nurse	Specific Examples of Nurse Communication
Verbal	
Nonverbal	

Next, let's look at an interaction between the nurse and a different patient.

- Click on **Leave the Floor** and then on **Restart the Program**.
- Sign in to work on the Skilled Nursing Floor for Period of Care 1.
- From the Patient List, select Kathryn Doyle (Room 503).
- Click on **Go to Nurses' Station** and then on **503** at the bottom of the screen.
- Click on **Patient Care** and then on **Nurse-Client Interactions**.
- Select and view the video titled **0730: Assessment—Biopsychosocial**. (*Note:* Check the virtual clock to see whether enough time has elapsed. You can use the fast-forward feature to advance the time by 2-minute intervals if the video is not yet available. Then click on **Patient Care** and **Nurse-Client Interactions** to refresh the screen.)

3. As you observe the 0730 video, make note of the therapeutic verbal and nonverbal communication techniques the nurse uses. Record these in the first column of the table below. Then, for each technique you identify, list specific examples of verbal and nonverbal communication used by the nurse that demonstrate the technique.

Therapeutic Communication Techniques Used by Nurse	Specific Examples of Nurse Communication
Verbal	
Nonverbal	

Understanding Responses to Stress

✐ **Reading Assignment:** Understanding Responses to Stress (Chapter 11)

Patient: Kelly Brady, Obstetrics Floor, Room 203

Goal: Care for a patient with both medical and psychiatric illness, using holistic approaches to manage the patient's stress.

Objectives:

- Describe the fight-or-flight response to stress.
- Describe the role of the sympathetic nervous system in the fight-or-flight response.
- Differentiate between eustress and distress.
- Identify factors that affect a patient's response to stress.
- Identify effective stress reduction techniques and their benefits.
- Identify the predisposing and precipitating stressors of the patient.
- Evaluate the significance of the patient's stressors.
- Determine the patient's coping resources and coping styles.
- Identify the patient's stage of treatment and implement corresponding nursing interventions.

Exercise 1

 Clinical Preparation: Writing Activity

 30 minutes

1. Define the fight-or-flight response to stress.

This is the body's way of preparing for a situation, an individual perceives as a threat to survival. It results in ↑BP, ↑HR, and ↑CO.

2. In the acute stress (alarm) stage of the general adaptation syndrome (GAS), three principal stress mediators are involved. Match them with their action.

Sympathetic Nervous System Part	Role in the Response to Stress
_C_ Brain cortex and hypothalamus	a. Sends messages to the adrenal cortex
_a_ Hypothalamus	b. Produces corticosteroids to increase muscle endurance and stamina
_b_ Adrenal cortex	c. Signals adrenal glands to release catecholamine adrenalin that increases heart rate, respirations, and blood pressure to enhance strength and speed

3. One's body reacts to positive and negative stress in the same way. Lazarus defined positive stress as eustress and negative stress as distress. Identify each of the following specific stressors as positive or negative.

Stressor	Type of Stressor
_b_ Wedding	a. Distress
_a_ Pain	b. Eustress
_a_ New baby	
_a b_ Breakup of a relationship	
_a b_ Hunger	
_a b_ Fear of terrorist attack	
_b_ Buying a car	

4. Factors such as age, sex, culture, life experiences, and lifestyle affect a patient's response to stress. Place an X next to each true statement below.

   _X_ Strong social support can act as a buffer against stress.

   _X_ Members of many cultures express distress in somatic terms.

   ____ Spiritual practices can weaken the immune system.

   ____ Women assess their own stress to be higher than that of men.

   _X_ Proper diet and exercise can help manage stress.

5. List four known benefits of stress reduction techniques.

- Sleep
- Exercise
- Reduction or Cessation of caffeine Intake
- Music
- Pets
- Message

6. Cognitive-behavioral techniques are the most effective methods to reduce stress. Match each of the following specific techniques with its type of method.

Specific Technique	Type of Method
__b__ Relaxation exercises	a. Behavioral (body)
__a__ Breathing exercises	b. Cognitive (mind)
__b__ Journal writing	
__b__ Reframing	
__b__ Meditation	
__a__ Humor	
__b__ Biofeedback	
__b__ Mindfulness	
__b__ Guided imagery	
__b__ Assertiveness and problem-solving training	
__a__ Physical exercise	

Exercise 2

 CD-ROM Activity

 30 minutes

- Sign in to work at Pacific View Regional Hospital on the Obstetrics Floor for Period of Care 3. (*Note:* If you are already in the virtual hospital from a previous exercise, click on **Leave the Floor** and then **Restart the Program** to get to the sign-in window.)
- From the Patient List, select Kelly Brady (Room 203).
- Click on **Go to Nurses' Station**.
- Click on **Chart** and then on **203**.
- Click on **Nursing Admission**.

1. In the Nursing Admission, the aspect of Kelly Brady's history that indicates she has

   had mental health problems in the past is _____.

2. The three recent stressful life events that might contribute to Kelly Brady's depression and

   anxiety are _____,

   _____, and

   _____.

3. How does Kelly Brady physically express her depression?

    a. Cries often and does not want to be alone
    b. Does not show her sadness
    c. Rocks back and forth
    d. Talks with friends

4. According to the Nursing Admission, Kelly Brady's main coping mechanism is

    _____.

5. How does Kelly Brady feel about her hospitalization?

- Click on **Return to Nurses' Station** and then on **203** at the bottom of your screen.
- Inside the patient's room, click on **Patient Care** and then on **Nurse-Client Interactions**.
- Select and view the video titled **1500: Transfer to Labor and Delivery**. (*Note:* Check the virtual clock to see whether enough time has elapsed. You can use the fast-forward feature to advance the time by 2-minute intervals if the video is not yet available. Then click on **Patient Care** and **Nurse-Client Interactions** to refresh the screen.)

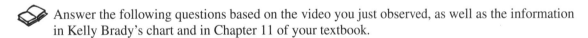

Answer the following questions based on the video you just observed, as well as the information in Kelly Brady's chart and in Chapter 11 of your textbook.

6. In terms of Hans Selye's general adaptation syndrome, what is Kelly Brady's treatment stage?

    a. Acute
    b. Prolonged

7. Given Kelly Brady's stage of treatment, identify the nurse's goal, assessment focus, purpose of interventions, and expected outcomes below.

Nursing goal

Focus of assessment

Purpose of intervention(s)

Expected outcome

8. During the video interaction, the action the nurse takes to indicate she is focusing on the

overall goal of stabilization is _____

_____

_____.

9. In the same interaction, the nurse educates Kelly Brady on the risk factors that are

threatening her health and well-being by _____.

10. The nurse attempts to manage the environment to provide safety for Kelly Brady by

_____.

LESSON 5

Anxiety and Anxiety Disorders

/OʘʘO **Reading Assignment:** Anxiety and Anxiety Disorders (Chapter 12)

Patient: Dorothy Grant, Obstetrics Floor, Room 201

Goal: To care for a pregnant patient who is experiencing anxiety.

Objectives:

- Define anxiety and describe its essential characteristics.
- Understand levels of anxiety.
- Describe physiological responses to anxiety.
- Define cognitive, behavioral, and affective responses to anxiety.
- Identify stressors leading to a patient's anxiety.
- Define defense mechanism.
- Identify effective medications prescribed for patients with anxiety.
- Discuss levels of anxiety as they relate to nursing interventions.
- Develop treatment interventions and outcomes for a patient with anxiety.
- Identify the characteristics of generalized anxiety disorder and posttraumatic stress disorder.

Exercise 1

Clinical Preparation: Writing Activity

30 minutes

1. _____Anxiety_____ is defined as a universal human experience that produces a diffuse, vague feeling of apprehension, including feelings of uneasiness, uncertainty, or dread.

2. Anxiety is experienced at different levels. Match each level of anxiety with its characteristics.

Level		Characteristic
_c_	Mild	a. The person may demonstrate selective inattention. As the perceptual field narrows, the person focuses on immediate concerns.
_a_	Moderate	
_d_	Severe	b. Associated with dread and terror, the person exhibits markedly disturbed behavior as the personality becomes disorganized.
_b_	Panic	
		c. Associated with tensions of daily life and may produce slight discomfort.
		d. Significant reduction in the perceptual field as the person focuses on specific or scattered details and cannot think of anything else. Learning and problem solving are not possible.

3. Identify at least two physiological responses to anxiety in each of the systems below and on the next page.

System	Physiological Response (Symptoms)
Cardiovascular	Tachycardia ↑ pulse rate
Respiratory	↑ respiratory rate ↑ in voice pitch hyperventilation

System	Physiological Response
Gastrointestinal	Urinary frequency Urinary urgency
Somatic (sensory)	headache backache Insomnia
Genitourinary tract	frequency urgency
Somatic (muscular)	↑ muscle tension foot tapping lip chewing

4. Match each type of anxiety disorder with its characteristics.

Characteristics

   _b_   Persistent reexperiencing of a highly traumatic event

   _a_   Excessive worry about numerous things lasting longer than 6 months

   _b_   Symptoms beginning within 3 months after the trauma

   _a_   Anxiety level out of proportion to the true impact of the event

   _a_   Persistent stimuli avoidance and numbing of general responsiveness

   _a_   Decision making difficult because of poor concentration and fear of making mistakes

Type of Anxiety Disorder

a. Generalized anxiety disorder (GAD)

b. Posttraumatic stress disorder (PTSD)

5. __Defense mechanisms__ protect people from painful awareness of feelings and memories that can provoke overwhelming anxiety.

6. Discuss three overall guidelines for basic nursing interventions in working with a patient with anxiety.

7. For patients with moderate to severe anxiety, medication may be a necessary intervention. In the table below, list the positive aspects and the cautions associated with the use of antidepressant and anxiolytic medications in patients with anxiety.

Medication Class	Positive Aspects	Cautions
Antidepressants (SSRIs)	* first-line tx for acute stress disorders and PTSD * rapid onset of action * fewer problematic side effects	- Do not ↑ dose or frequency of injestion without prior approval of therapist - These medication ↓ the ability to handle mechanical equipment (e.g., cars, saws, and machinery)
Anxiolytics (Antianxiety agents)	* used to treat the somatic and psychological symptoms	- Do not drink alcoholic beverages or take other antianxiety drugs, because depressant effects of both would be potentiated - To avoid drinking beverages containing caffeine, because they decrease the desired effects of the drug - Potential for dependence

Exercise 2

  CD-ROM Activity

30 minutes

- Sign in to work at Pacific View Regional Hospital on the Obstetrics Floor for Period of Care 1. (*Note:* If you are already in the virtual hospital from a previous exercise, click on **Leave the Floor** and then **Restart the Program** to get to the sign-in window.)
- From the Patient List, select Dorothy Grant (Room 201).
- Click on **Get Report**.

1. According to the change-of-shift report, what level of anxiety is Dorothy Grant experiencing?

   a. Mild
   b. Moderate
   c. Severe
   d. Panic

2. It is reported that Dorothy Grant's stated concerns of _____

   and the _____ are causing her anxiety.

 • Now click on **Go to Nurses' Station** and then on **201** at the bottom of your screen.
- Click on **Patient Care** and then on **Nurse-Client Interactions**.
- Select and view the video titled **0730: Patient Teaching—Medication**. (*Note:* Check the virtual clock to see whether enough time has elapsed. You can use the fast-forward feature to advance the time by 2-minute intervals if the video is not yet available. Then click on **Patient Care** and **Nurse-Client Interactions** to refresh the screen.)

3. How does the nurse's assessment of Dorothy Grant's anxiety level compare with assessment contained in the change-of-shift report?

→ • Now click on **Chart** and then on **201**.
   • Read the **Nursing Admission** record.

4. What are the two stressors listed that contribute to Dorothy Grant's anxiety?

5. Dorothy Grant is experiencing traumatic injury by her husband. What is your reaction (thoughts and feelings) to this event as a reason for the patient's anxiety?

6. Dorothy Grant has been using maladaptive coping mechanisms to handle her stressors. For each unhealthy coping mechanism listed in the table below and on the next page, identify an alternative healthy coping mechanism.

Unhealthy Coping Mechanism	Healthy Coping Mechanism
Hoping the abuse will stop	

Unhealthy Coping Mechanism	Healthy Coping Mechanism
Keeping the children quiet	
Blaming herself for causing the abuse (pregnancy)	
Trying not to upset husband	

7. You have assessed Dorothy Grant's level of anxiety to be moderate in severity. Develop nursing interventions based on the aspects of treatment listed below and on the next page.

Aspects	Nursing Interventions
Recognition	

Aspects	Nursing Interventions
Insight	
Education	
Coping	

→ • Click on **Return to Room 201**.
   • Click on **MAR** and review Dorothy Grant's medications.
   • Check to see whether there are any medications ordered for Dorothy Grant's anxiety.

8. What classification of medications would typically be ordered for a patient with moderate to severe anxiety?

   a. Stimulants
   b. Antidepressants
   c. Antipsychotics
   d. Antianxiety agents
   e. Both b and d

9. In deciding whether to order medication to treat Dorothy Grant's anxiety, what are the key considerations?

   a. 30 weeks pregnant/possible contraindications
   b. Anxiety initially assessed to be at a moderate level
   c. Blunt force trauma to abdomen/may result in preterm delivery
   d. Need more time to assess patient's anxiety level
   e. All of the above

10. The best treatment outcomes will demonstrate adaptive ways of coping with stress. From the list below, place an X next to the two treatment outcome statements that best describe desired outcomes based on Dorothy Grant's treatment plan.

   _____ Verbalizes need for assistance, seeks information, and modifies lifestyle as needed

   _____ Identifies and plans coping strategies for stressful situations

   _____ Monitors intensity of anxiety and maintains adequate sleep

   _____ Accepts compliments from others

Depressive Disorders

/Oᴦᴼ **Reading Assignment:** Depressive Disorders (Chapter 13)

Patient: Kelly Brady, Obstetrics Floor, Room 203

Goal: To care for a patient experiencing a medical health crisis who is also experiencing symptoms of depression.

Objectives:

- Understand prevalence of depression.
- Describe predisposing risk factors and precipitating stressors in depression.
- Assess a patient who is experiencing depression.
- Identify symptoms associated with depression.
- Discuss safety as it relates to the treatment of a patient with depression.
- Explore the recovery model of treatment.
- Understand the relationship between depression and pregnancy.
- Identify treatment phases of a patient with depression.
- Describe effective treatments including pharmacological treatment for depressed patients.
- Develop a treatment plan for a patient with depression.

Exercise 1

Clinical Preparation: Writing Activity

30 minutes

1. The lifetime prevalence of a major depressive episode is now 8.6%. Which of the following statements about depression is/are true?

    a. Major depressive disorders are twice as common in women as in men.
    b. Depression is the leading cause of disability in the United States.
    c. Major depressive and dysthymic disorders tend to have higher prevalence rates in lower income groups.
    d. Girls 15 years and older are twice as likely to have a major depressive episode as are boys.
    e. All of the above are true.

2. Depression may result from a complex interaction of causes and common risk factors for depression. Place an X next to all that apply.

    X   Negative stressful life events, especially loss and humiliation

    X   Female gender

    X   History of prior depressive episode(s)

    X   Alcohol/substance abuse

    X   Postpartum period

    X   Medical illnesses

    X   Lack of social support

    X   Family history of depressive disorders, especially in first-degree relatives

    X   History of suicidal attempts or a family history of same

3. Complete the table below and on the next page by listing symptoms associated with persons with depression.

Areas to Assess	Symptoms
Affect	– Facial expressions convey sadness and dejection – Crying – No eye contact – monotone – little or no facial expression

Areas to Assess	**Symptoms**
Thought processes	- Poor judgement - Poor memory - Poor concentration - delusional thinking
Mood/feelings	- anxiety - worthlessness - guilt - helplessness - hopelessness - anger
Physical behavior	- lethargy - fatigue - Δ in sleep pattern - Δ in bowel pattern - loss of libido

4. Approximately 15% of people with clinical depression commit suicide. In assessing patients with depression, it is important to think about safety first. Explain the actions the nurse will take to make sure the patient is safe.

5. The New Freedom Commission on Mental Illness (2003) stated that national health priorities should concentrate on recovery from mental illness including depression. Discuss the recovery model and list its characteristics.

6. There are three phases in the treatment of and the recovery from major depression. Match each phase with its associated interventions.

Interventions	Phases
_____ Directed at prevention of relapse	a. Acute
_____ Directed at reduction of depressive symptoms and restoration of psychosocial and work function; hospitalization may be required	b. Continuation
	c. Maintenance
_____ Directed at prevention of further episodes of depression	

7. Within the recovery model, health teaching is very important as it allows patients to make informed choices and can be used to provide hope. What should the nurse include in health teaching with a patient who is depressed?

8. Successful behavior is a powerful tool to counteract depression. Discuss specific interventions the nurse can make in caring for the depressed patient to effect positive behavioral change. Include three activities the patient can accomplish to make positive behavioral changes.

9. For treating patients with depression, which class of medication has proven the most effective with the least amount of side effects?

a. Selective serotonin reuptake inhibitors (SSRIs)
b. Monoamine oxidase inhibitors (MAOIs)
c. Tricyclic antidepressant drugs (TCAs)

Exercise 2

 CD-ROM Activity

 30 minutes

- Sign in to work at Pacific View Regional Hospital on the Obstetrics Floor for Period of Care 1. (*Note:* If you are already in the virtual hospital from a previous exercise, click on **Leave the Floor** and then **Restart the Program** to get to the sign-in window.)
- From the Patient List, select Kelly Brady (Room 203).
- Click on **Get Report** and review.
- Click on **Go to Nurses' Station** and then on **203** at the bottom of the screen.
- Now click on **Patient Care** and then on **Physical Assessment**.
- Click on **Head & Neck**.
- Select **Mental Status** (in the green boxes).

1. Based on the mental status assessment, Kelly Brady's two documented behavioral symptoms are _____ and _____.

2. Along with depression, Kelly Brady has anxiety, which is not uncommon. What percentage of the population is reported to have anxiety co-occurring with depression?

   a. 20%
   b. 50%
   c. 70%
   d. 90%

→ • Now click on **Chart** and then on **203**.
   • Click on **History and Physical** and review.

3. The predisposing factor in Kelly Brady's family history related to depression is

   _____. In her past medical

   history, the key fact related to depression is _____

   _____.

→ • Now click on **Nursing Admission** and review.

4. Given Kelly Brady's history and current life situation, how many risk factors does she have?

   a. 2
   b. 4
   c. 6
   d. 8

5. What are Kelly Brady's major life events/precipitating stressors that are contributing to her depression?

   a. Lack of support: Mother with cancer, parents out of town, and sister going through divorce
   b. Financial stress: Problems with her job and husband's job and moving into larger home
   c. Biological factors: Pregnancy
   d. All of the above

6. List all the behavioral symptoms Kelly Brady is experiencing related to depression.

7. To develop a treatment plan to address Kelly Brady's depression, complete the table below.

Area	Goal	Interventions
Environment/safety		
Cognitive		
Behavioral		
Social skills		
Education		

8. Discuss how Kelly Brady's pregnancy might be related to her depression.

9. Kelly Brady's physician states that he would recommend she take paroxetine after the birth of her baby. From the records you have read, complete the statements below.

The trade name for paroxetine is _____, and the dose that was recommended

was _____. One clinical rationale for recommending paroxetine is that

_____.

Schizophrenia

👓 **Reading Assignment:** Schizophrenia (Chapter 15)

Patient: Jacquline Catanazaro, Medical-Surgical Floor, Room 402

Goal: To care for a patient with chronic schizophrenia who is hospitalized for acute asthma.

Objectives:

- Define schizophrenia and its characteristics.
- Discuss the prevalence of schizophrenia.
- List the positive and negative symptoms of schizophrenia.
- Understand symptoms of schizophrenia and their impact on the cognitive, perceptual, emotional, behavioral, and socialization of the person.
- Identify predisposing factors and precipitating stressors of schizophrenia.
- Discuss the focus of treatment for each phase of the illness.
- Identify communication techniques the nurse uses for patients exhibiting the positive symptoms of hallucinations and delusions.
- Describe the importance of education as part of the treatment plan for a patient with schizophrenia.
- Explain the importance of relapse prevention for a patient with schizophrenia.
- Discuss medication as a treatment for patients diagnosed with schizophrenia.

Exercise 1

 Clinical Preparation: Writing Activity

15 minutes

1. _____ is a potentially devastating brain disorder that affects a person's thinking, language, emotions, social behavior, and ability to perceive reality accurately.

2. Schizophrenia is a psychotic disorder characterized by symptoms such as

   _____; _____; and disorganized

   _____, _____, and/or _____.

3. The impact of schizophrenia on the individual and society is enormous. Place an X next to each true statement about schizophrenia.

   _____ Schizophrenia affects 1 in every 100 people in the United States.

   _____ Men and women are equally represented in the population of individuals with schizophrenia.

   _____ Of people diagnosed with schizophrenia, 100% have the disease for life.

   _____ The most typical onset of schizophrenia is between the ages of 18 and 25.

   _____ Only 10% of those with schizophrenia have nicotine dependence.

   _____ Substance abuse disorders occur in approximately 50% of individuals with schizophrenia.

   _____ Almost 50% of patients with schizophrenia attempt suicide.

4. It is important to understand the positive and negative symptoms of schizophrenia. List the positive and negative symptoms associated with schizophrenia.

Positive Symptoms	**Negative Symptoms**

5. Many stressors or triggers often precede a new episode or exacerbation of the symptoms of schizophrenia. Match the specific trigger to its corresponding category.

Common Relapse Trigger	**Category of Stressor**
_____ Low self-concept/self-confidence	a. Health
_____ Lack of social support	b. Environment
_____ Housing difficulties	c. Attitudes
_____ Aggressive/violent behavior	d. Behavior
_____ Lack of sleep	
_____ Poor medication management	
_____ Lack of transportation	
_____ Financial problems	
_____ Job pressures	
_____ Poor nutrition	
_____ Social isolation	
_____ Interpersonal difficulties	

6. The three phases of treatment for schizophrenia are acute, maintenance, and stabilization. Place an X next to any of the following that reflect the focus during the acute phase of treatment.

_____ Limit setting

_____ Adaptation to deficits

_____ Psychopharmacological treatment in crisis

_____ Medication teaching and side effect management

_____ Crisis intervention

_____ Cognitive and social skill enhancement

_____ Safety assessment

_____ Family support groups

_____ Symptom stabilization

7. Communicating with a patient who has schizophrenia can be challenging. In the table below, list three communication techniques that may be helpful with patients experiencing the positive symptoms of hallucinations and delusions.

Positive Symptom	Communication Techniques
Hallucinations	
Delusions	

8. The course of schizophrenia usually includes recurrent and acute exacerbations of psychosis. Discuss the role of preventing relapse in treating patients with schizophrenia.

Exercise 2

 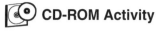 **CD-ROM Activity**

45 minutes

- Sign in to work at Pacific View Regional Hospital on the Medical-Surgical Floor for Period of Care 3. (*Note:* If you are already in the virtual hospital from a previous exercise, click on **Leave the Floor** and then **Restart the Program** to get to the sign-in window.)
- From the Patient List, select Jacquline Catanazaro (Room 402).
- Click on **Go to Nurses' Station**.
- Click on **Chart** and then on **402**.
- Click on **Nurse's Notes**.
- Read the admission note for Monday at 1600.

1. Identify two pieces of information contained in the nurse's admission note that have implications for discharge planning.

    a. Patient has asthma.
    b. Sister is patient's main support.
    c. Patient has no transportation.
    d. Patient has a history of stopping her psychiatric medication.
    e. Both b and d.

 • Now read the Nurse's Notes dated Tuesday at 0400.

2. The statement made by Jacquline Catanazaro that people are putting poison into her IV is an example of what type of delusion?

    a. Grandiose
    b. Persecutory
    c. Paranoid
    d. None of the above

• Now read the Nurse's Notes dated Wednesday at 0600.

3. The note describes symptoms of schizophrenia that have a direct relationship to Jacquline Catanazaro's asthma. Explain the relationship.

➔ • Now click on **Consultation**.
   • Read the Psychiatric Consult.

4. The positive symptom of schizophrenia described in the report is

   _____. The negative symptoms described are

   _____ and _____.

5. The plan contained within the Psychiatric Consult includes exercise and nutrition.
   Comment on the relevance of diet and exercise as part of the plan of care for this patient.

→ • Click on **History and Physical** and review.
 • Next, click on **Nursing Admission**.

6. Relapse can be a devastating part of the disease of schizophrenia. For each category below and on the next page, list Jacquline Catanazaro's barriers to compliance that may result in future relapses.

Category	Barriers to Compliance
Health	
Thoughts	
Attitudes	

Category	Barriers to Compliance
Behavior	
Socialization	
Medication	

7. Education will be a critical component of Jacquline Catanazaro's treatment plan. Place an X next to each of her educational needs.

_____ Healthy living

_____ Medication

_____ Psychoeducation

_____ Illness management

• Click on **Return to Nurses' Station** and then on **402** at the bottom of the screen.
- Click on **Patient Care** and then on **Nurse-Client Interactions**.
- Select and view the video titled **1500: Intervention—Patient Teaching**.
- Now select and view the video titled **1540: Discharge Planning**. (*Note:* Check the virtual clock to see whether enough time has elapsed. You can use the fast-forward feature to advance the time by 2-minute intervals if the video is not yet available. Then click on **Patient Care** and **Nurse-Client Interactions** to refresh the screen.)

8. Discuss the importance of including the patient's sister in the discharge planning and relapse prevention process.

• Click on **MAR** and then on tab **402**.
- Scroll down to locate the antipsychotic medication ordered.
- Click on **Return to Room 402**.
- Click on the **Drug** icon and look up the medication you found in the MAR.

9. Using the Drug Guide, complete the information specified below and on the next page for the antipsychotic medication ordered for Jacquline Catanazaro.

Name of medication

Indication

Mechanism of action

Side effects

Dosage

Nursing considerations

Patient teaching

10. Consider the medication dosage Jacquline Catanazaro is receiving and the usual dosage out-
    lined in the Drug Guide. What might be the rationale for the current dosage the physician is
    giving to this patient?

Eating Disorders

✐ **Reading Assignment:** Eating Disorders (Chapter 16)

Patient: Tiffany Sheldon, Pediatrics Floor, Room 305

Goal: To provide nursing care for a patient with an eating disorder who also has comorbid psychiatric symptoms.

Objectives:

- Discuss the prevalence of eating disorders.
- Identify common symptoms of eating disorders.
- Identify the predisposing factors related to eating disorders.
- List psychological problems and serious medical complications associated with eating disorders.
- Apply the nursing process in caring for a patient with an eating disorder.
- Assess interactions between the nurse and a patient with an eating disorder.
- Identify coping resources and coping mechanisms related to eating disorders.
- Develop a treatment plan for a patient with an eating disorder.
- List outcomes for a patient with an eating disorder.

Exercise 1

 Clinical Preparation: Writing Activity

15 minutes

1. Food is essential to life because it nourishes the body and soul, but to someone who feels

    his or her life is out of control, it can be used to _____.

2. The prevalence of eating disorders is on the increase in our culture. In addition, comorbid psychiatric illnesses are high in patients with eating disorders. Place an X next to each true statement regarding eating disorder statistics.

    _____ The rate of eating disorders among middle-aged women has increased with the baby boomer generation.

    _____ Eating disorders are more common among men than among women.

    _____ Most eating disorders begin in the early teens to mid-20s.

    _____ Incidence of obsessive-compulsive disorders has been reported as high as 25% in those with eating disorders, most common in those with anorexia nervosa.

    _____ The major cause of death in patients diagnosed with eating disorders is suicide.

    _____ Depression and anxiety are common comorbid conditions in people with all types of eating disorders.

    _____ A history of sexual abuse is less common in those with eating disorders than in the general population.

    _____ Fewer than 50% of people with eating disorders seek medical care.

3. Place an X next to the statements that best reflect the most common symptoms of eating disorders.

    _____ Intense fear of gaining weight

    _____ Skipping meals occasionally

    _____ Depriving self of needed nourishment

    _____ Severe dieting

    _____ Overeating under stress

    _____ Chewing food very slowly

    _____ Frequent fasting

    _____ Binge eating behaviors

    _____ Thinking of oneself as fat even though underweight

    _____ Self-induced vomiting

4. Disordered eating can lead to serious medical and psychological complications. List the complications in the table below.

Medical Complications	Psychological Problems

5. How do sociocultural factors regarding body size affect the prevalence of eating disorders in women?

6. There are many factors that predispose a person to develop an eating disorder. Place an X next to the predisposing factors associated with eating disorders.

_____ Rigid, meticulous, ritualistic, obsessive-compulsive behaviors

_____ No early childhood issues and a healthy family life

_____ Pervasive sense of ineffectiveness and helplessness; no control over life

_____ Understanding others' feelings and being able to handle one's own intense emotions

_____ Cognitive distortions

_____ History of sexual abuse

7. Many people who are in treatment for eating disorders have evidence of other psychiatric disorders. Complete the psychiatric comorbidity for each eating disorder listed in the table below.

Eating Disorder	Psychiatric Comorbidity
Anorexia nervosa	
Bulimia nervosa	
Binge eating disorder	

8. Discuss the environmental factors that may predispose someone to an eating disorder.

9. What sociocultural biases do you have regarding those who have eating disorders that result in them being severely underweight or overweight?

Exercise 2

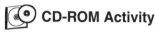 **CD-ROM Activity**

 15 minutes

- Sign in to work at Pacific View Regional Hospital on the Pediatrics Floor for Period of Care 1. (*Note:* If you are already in the virtual hospital from a previous exercise, click on **Leave the Floor** and then **Restart the Program** to get to the sign-in window.)
- From the Patient List, select Tiffany Sheldon (Room 305).
- Click on **Get Report** and review.
- Click on **Go to Nurses' Station**.
- Click on **305** at the bottom of your screen and read the **Initial Observations**.

1. Behaviors Tiffany is exhibiting that may be indicative of comorbid psychiatric disorders

   are _____, _____, and

   _____.

➡ - Click on **Patient Care** and then on **Physical Assessment**.
- Click on **Head & Neck**.
- Click on **Mental Status** (in the green boxes).

2. Place an X next to each finding from the mental status assessment that coincides with the shift report and initial observations.

   _____ Good eye contact

   _____ Listless

   _____ Flat affect

   _____ Energetic

   _____ Avoids eye contact

   _____ Withdrawn

➡ - Click on **Patient Care** and then on **Nurse-Client Interactions**.
- Select and view the video titled **0730: Initial Assessment**. (*Note:* Check the virtual clock to see whether enough time has elapsed. You can use the fast-forward feature to advance the time by 2-minute intervals if the video is not yet available. Then click on **Patient Care** and **Nurse-Client Interactions** to refresh the screen.)

3. Describe your reaction to Tiffany Sheldon's responses to the nurse who is caring for her.

➡ • Click on **Chart** and then on **305**.
   • Click on **Physician's Orders**.

4. In addition to the physical assessment, which of the following orders indicate that multi-disciplinary assessments are being implemented for Tiffany Sheldon's care?

   a. Nursing supervision during and after meals
   b. Nutritionist to follow patient
   c. Include Adolescent Care Team
   d. Involve Eating Disorders Clinic
   e. Consult with Psychiatric Team
   f. All of the above

➡ • Click on **History and Physical** and review.

5. Tiffany Sheldon's medical diagnoses are _____,

_____, and _____.

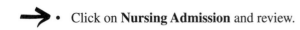 • Click on **Nursing Admission** and review.

6. List at least two possible psychological and two environmental predisposing factors associated with Tiffany Sheldon's eating disorder.

• Click on **Return to Room 305** to exit the chart.

Exercise 3

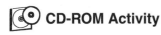 **CD-ROM Activity**

 30 minutes

- Sign in to work at Pacific View Regional Hospital on the Pediatrics Floor for Period of Care 3. (*Note:* If you are already in the virtual hospital from a previous exercise, click on **Leave the Floor** and then **Restart the Program** to get to the sign-in window.)
- From the Patient List, select Tiffany Sheldon (Room 305).
- Click on **Go to Nurses' Station** and then on **305** at the bottom of your screen.
- Click on **Patient Care** and then on **Nurse-Client Interactions**.
- Select and view the video titled **1500: Relapse—Contributing Factors**. (*Note:* Check the virtual clock to see whether enough time has elapsed. You can use the fast-forward feature to advance the time by 2-minute intervals if the video is not yet available. Then click on **Patient Care** and **Nurse-Client Interactions** to refresh the screen.)

1. Tiffany Sheldon's predisposing factors make her especially vulnerable to environmental pressures and stress. Choose the stressors that have contributed to the current relapse of her eating disorder.

   a. Parents divorced 3 years ago
   b. Family does not understand her problem
   c. Mom is angry and "disgusted"
   d. Visited Dad in Florida 2 weeks ago
   e. Both c and d

 • Click on **Chart** and then on **305**.
- Click on **Mental Health**.
- Read the Psychiatric/Mental Health Assessment.

2. Characteristic of those who have anorexia, Tiffany Sheldon's main maladaptive coping

   mechanism is _____.

3. For people with anorexia, the issue is not really their weight, but rather their control over their own life and fears. An example of this overriding concern occurs when Tiffany

   Sheldon states, "_____."

4. In addition to Tiffany Sheldon's nursing diagnosis of *Imbalanced nutrition, less than body requirements*, identify two nursing diagnoses that best describe the psychological components to her eating disorder.

 • Click on **Return to Room 305**.
 • Click on **Patient Care** and then on **Nurse-Client Interactions**.
 • Select and view the video titled **1530: Facilitating Success**. (*Note:* Check the virtual clock to see whether enough time has elapsed. You can use the fast-forward feature to advance the time by 2-minute intervals if the video is not yet available. Then click on **Patient Care** and **Nurse-Client Interactions** to refresh the screen.)

5. One of the most important aspects in assessing patients with an eating disorder is their motivation to change their behavior. What statement does Tiffany Sheldon make that would best define her motivation level? Discuss the impact her motivational level will have in preventing relapse.

- Click on **Chart** and then on **305**.
- Click on **Consultations**.
- Read the Psychiatric Consult.

6. Tiffany Sheldon has two simultaneous plans of care being implemented. One plan involves the eating contract, and the other is the plan devised as a result of the Psychiatric Consult. Complete the table below and on the next page by identifying interventions for each element of the psychosocial treatment plan.

Psychosocial Treatment Plan	Specific Interventions
Individual therapy	
Family conference/family therapy	

Psychosocial Treatment Plan	**Specific Interventions**

Relationship to eating contract

Medication

 • Still in the chart, click on **Patient Education**.
• Read the report.

7. Identify the treatment outcomes for Tiffany. Can you think of other important outcomes?

Cognitive Disorders

Reading Assignment: Cognitive Disorders (Chapter 17)

Patient: Carlos Reyes, Skilled Nursing Floor, Room 504

Goal: To care for a patient who has cognitive impairment and symptoms of cardiovascular disease.

Objectives:

- Compare and contrast characteristics of delirium, dementia, and amnestic disorders.
- Provide examples of severe disturbed behavior associated with dementia.
- Understand underlying principles of nursing interventions for patients with cognitive impairment.
- Discuss nursing interventions in working with patients with delirium and dementia.
- Identify underlying medical conditions that can produce symptoms of delirium.
- Identify medications used in the treatment of dementia and agitation.
- Discuss the importance of family involvement in discharge planning and home care.

Exercise 1

 Clinical Preparation: Writing Activity

15 minutes

1. It is important to distinguish between dementia and delirium because a delayed or missed diagnosis can have serious complications and the greater the risk for

   _____.

2. It is important to distinguish among the cognitive disorders of delirium, dementia, and amnestic disorder. Match the following characteristics with their corresponding disorder.

   Characteristics   **Disorder**

   _____ Develops slowly; multiple cognitive deficits   a. Delirium
           including impairment in memory without
           impairment in consciousness; progressive.   b. Dementia
           Majority are irreversible.
                                                                      c. Amnestic disorder
   _____ Loss in both short- and long-term memory in
           absence of other cognitive impairments;
           always secondary to underlying causes.

   _____ Disturbance in consciousness and change in
           cognition developed over short period of time;
           always secondary to another condition.

3. In addition to the usual dementia symptoms of disorientation, confusion, memory loss, disorganized thinking, and poor judgment, a considerable number of individuals with dementia have secondary behavioral disturbances, including depression, hallucinations, delusions, agitation, insomnia, and wandering. Match each of the following examples to its category.

   Behavior Category   **Examples of Behavior**

   _____ Aggressive psychomotor behavior   a. Incontinence, poor hygiene

   _____ Nonaggressive psychomotor   b. Demanding, complaining, screaming,
           behavior   disruptive

   _____ Verbally aggressive behavior   c. Decreased activity, apathy, withdrawal,
                                                     depression
   _____ Passive behavior
                                                  d. Hitting, kicking, pushing, scratching,
   _____ Functionally impaired behavior   assault

   _____ Other thought disorders   e. Restlessness, pacing, wandering

                                                  f. Hallucinations, delusions

4. Nursing interventions for cognitively impaired patients focus on:

   a. protecting patient's dignity.
   b. preserving functional status.
   c. promoting quality of life.
   d. all of the above.

5. Any major imbalance of body functions can disrupt cognitive functioning. Discuss cardiac disorders and cardiac medications as potential precipitating stressors in delirium.

6. In caring for the patient experiencing symptoms of delirium, priority is given to nursing

   interventions that _____. Three nursing interventions that maintain life

   are _____,

   _____, and

   _____.

7. Planning the care for a patient with dementia is geared toward the patient's

   _____ needs. The single most effective tool in caring for patients with

   dementia is the nurse's attitude of _____.

8. In providing care to patients with dementia, priority is given to nursing interventions that maintain the patient's optimum level of functioning. With that in mind, complete the table below and on the next page by listing nursing interventions for each component of care.

Component of Care	Interventions
Social interaction	
Medications	
Orientation	
Communication	

Component of Care	Interventions
Wandering	
Agitation	
Family and community	

Exercise 2

 CD-ROM Activity

 15 minutes

- Sign in to work at Pacific View Regional Hospital on the Skilled Nursing Floor for Period of Care 2. (*Note:* If you are already in the virtual hospital from a previous exercise, click on **Leave the Floor** and then **Restart the Program** to get to the sign-in window.)
- From the Patient List, select Carlos Reyes (Room 504).
- Click on **Get Report**.
- Read both shift reports.

1. Based on the shift reports, Carlos Reyes' most problematic symptoms have been

   _____,

   _____, and

   _____.

 • Now click on **Go to Nurses' Station**.
- Click on Room **504** at the bottom of the screen.
- Click on **Patient Care** and then on **Physical Assessment**.
- Click on **Head & Neck**.
- Select **Mental Status** (in the green boxes).

2. From the mental status assessment, what symptoms indicate that Carlos Reyes is having cognitive impairments?

3. In the list below, place an X next to each behavior Carlos Reyes is exhibiting that is associated with aggression.

_____   Extreme anxiety

_____   Irritability

_____   Soft-spoken voice

_____   Confusion

_____   Intact memory

_____   Disorientation

 • Now click on **Patient Care** and then on **Nurse-Client Interactions**.

• Select and view the video titled **1120: The Agitated Patient**. (*Note:* Check the virtual clock to see whether enough time has elapsed. You can use the fast-forward feature to advance the time by 2-minute intervals if the video is not yet available. Then click on **Patient Care** and **Nurse-Client Interactions** to refresh the screen.)

4. Which intervention(s) did the nurse use to respond to Carlos Reyes' agitation?

   a. Ignored the difficult behavior
   b. Listened to the patient and patient's daughter
   c. Spoke in a calm, reassuring manner to decrease stress in the environment
   d. Modified the original plan to meet the patient's needs
   e. Did all except a

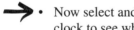 • Now select and view the video titled **1140: Assessing for Referrals**. (*Note:* Check the virtual clock to see whether enough time has elapsed. You can use the fast-forward feature to advance the time by 2-minute intervals if the video is not yet available. Then click on **Patient Care** and **Nurse-Client Interactions** to refresh the screen.)

5. Assess the son's understanding of Carlos Reyes' illness. What action will the nurse need to take after her brief interaction with the patient's son?

Exercise 3

 CD-ROM Activity

 30 minutes

- Sign in to work at Pacific View Regional Hospital on the Skilled Nursing Floor for Period of Care 3. (*Note:* If you are already in the virtual hospital from a previous exercise, click on **Leave the Floor** and then **Restart the Program** to get to the sign-in window.)
- From the Patient List, select Carlos Reyes (Room 504).
- Click on **Go to Nurses' Station**.
- Click on **Chart** and then on **504**.
- Read the **History and Physical** and review.
- Read the **Nursing Admission** and review.

1. Based on your review of all the pertinent data, what factors may be contributing to Carlos Reyes' confusion? Select all that apply.

    _____ Change in environment

    _____ Recent MI

    _____ History of dementia

    _____ Medication regimen

2. If Carlos Reyes returns to his daughter's home after discharge, discuss the problems that his daughter may have in caring for him.

• Click on **Return to Nurses' Station** and then on **504** at the bottom of the screen.
- Click on **Patient Care** and then on **Nurse-Client Interactions**.
- Select and view the video titled **1500: The Confused Patient**.
- Next, select and view the video titled **1505: Family Teaching—Dementia**. (*Note:* Check the virtual clock to see whether enough time has elapsed. You can use the fast-forward feature to advance the time by 2-minute intervals if the video is not yet available. Then click on **Patient Care** and **Nurse-Client Interactions** to refresh the screen.)

3. Describe the approach the nurse used in dealing with Carlos Reyes' confusion.

4. Interventions that involve family members of patients with dementia are critical to the success of the discharge plan. In the interaction with Carlos Reyes' daughter at 1505, what intervention did the nurse use?

 • Click on **MAR** and then on tab **504**.
- Find the medication ordered for anxiety and agitation.
- Click on **Return to Room 504** and then click on the **Drug** icon in the bottom left corner of the screen.
- Locate and review the medication you identified in the MAR.

5. Below and on the next page, provide the information requested for the drug ordered for Carlos Reyes' anxiety and agitation.

Generic name of medication

Class

Mechanism of action

Therapeutic effect

Indication

Dosage

Side effects

Nursing indications

 • Click on **Return to Room 504**.

- Click on **Patient Care** and then on **Nurse-Client Interactions**.

- Select and view the video titled **1525: Family Conflict—Discharge Plan**. (*Note:* Check the virtual clock to see whether enough time has elapsed. You can use the fast-forward feature to advance the time by 2-minute intervals if the video is not yet available. Then click on **Patient Care** and **Nurse-Client Interactions** to refresh the screen.)

- Now click on **Chart** and then on **504**.

- Click on **Consultations**.

- Read the Discharge Coordinator Consult.

6. Describe the family conflict associated with Carlos Reyes' care and its importance in planning for discharge. Also describe how the nurse should best approach the family situation.

7. Support for Carlos Reyes' family members will be crucial for their caretaking role. Given the patient's illness and family situation, list the types of community support that will be most beneficial.

8. In successful discharge planning, practical recommendations are necessary for family members who must care for patients with dementia, especially those who are also agitated and demonstrate aggressive behavior. In thinking about what you know about Carlos Reyes, provide some practical approaches below that you would recommend to his daughter.

Area of Focus	Practical Approaches
Environment	
Communication	
Self-care basics	

Addictive Disorders

📖 **Reading Assignment:** Addictive Disorders (Chapter 18)

Patient: Laura Wilson, Obstetrics Floor, Room 206

Goal: To care for a patient with acute medical needs who also has a diagnosis of polysubstance abuse.

Objectives:

- Discuss the prevalence of drug use in the United States.
- Understand terms associated with addictive disorders.
- Identify risks associated with a drug use lifestyle.
- Examine your own feelings about working with patients who have polysubstance abuse and who are HIV-positive and pregnant.
- Identify precipitating stressors, coping mechanisms, and resources of a patient with polysubstance abuse.
- Identify categories to include in an assessment of a patient with polysubstance abuse.
- Identify key aspects of the treatment plan for patients with polysubstance abuse.
- Discuss critical elements of discharge planning for patients who have substance abuse.

Exercise 1

 Clinical Preparation: Writing Activity

15 minutes

1. Cocaine, a drug that acts on the dopamine system in the brain and creates pleasurable

   changes in mental and emotional states, has the greatest potential for _____.

2. The prevalence of drug use in the United States is high. Place an X next to each true statement about drug use.

   _____ Approximately 18% of the U.S. population will abuse alcohol, and 13% will become dependent on alcohol.

   _____ Marijuana is the most widely used illicit drug in the United States.

   _____ Cocaine abusers may experience extreme weight loss and malnutrition, myocardial infarction, and stroke.

   _____ About 50% of full-time college students binge drink or use substances on a monthly basis.

   _____ When crack is smoked, it takes 4 to 6 seconds to take effect.

3. When discussing drug use, terms of abuse are important to understand. Match each term with its corresponding definition.

Term	**Definition**
_____ Substance abuse	a. Usually moderate to severe physical symptoms when substances are stopped
_____ Substance dependence	
_____ Addiction	b. The coexistence of substance abuse and a psychiatric disorder
_____ Co-occurring disorders	c. Includes withdrawal symptoms and tolerance to substance
_____ Physical dependence	
_____ Withdrawal symptoms	d. Continued use of substances despite related problems
_____ Tolerance	e. Loss of control of substance consumption; continued use despite associated problems; tendency to relapse
	f. Result from a biological need that occurs when the body becomes used to having the substance in the system
	g. Physiological reaction to a drug decreases with repeated administrations of the same dose

4. Discuss the importance of drug toxicology testing of patients who present with symptoms of possible substance abuse.

5. Lifestyles associated with substance abuse carry risks. Which of the following lifestyle risks is/are associated with substance abuse?

   a. Accidents
   b. Violence
   c. Self-neglect
   d. Physical and mental illnesses
   e. Complications during pregnancy
   f. Fetal abnormalities and substance dependence
   g. Hepatitis B and C
   h. HIV and AIDS
   i. All of the above

6. The nurse can detect current alcohol and other drug problems by asking two questions that are easily incorporated into the clinical interview. List the two questions below.

Exercise 2

 CD-ROM Activity

 15 minutes

- Sign in to work at Pacific View Regional Hospital on the Obstetrics Floor for Period of Care 1. (*Note:* If you are already in the virtual hospital from a previous exercise, click on **Leave the Floor** and then **Restart the Program** to get to the sign-in window.)
- From the Patient List, select Laura Wilson (Room 206).
- Click on **Go to Nurses' Station**.
- Click on **Chart** and then on **206**.
- Click on **Emergency Department** and read the report.

1. What information alerts the nurse that Laura Wilson may be abusing drugs?

    a. Found unconscious
    b. Nausea and diarrhea
    c. HIV-positive
    d. History of drug abuse
    e. a and d only

2. The assessment of chemical impairment is becoming more complex because of the increase in the simultaneous use of many substances (polydrug abuse). Laura Wilson's urine drug toxicology screen came back positive for THC (marijuana) and cocaine. Complete the table below and on the next page regarding the characteristics of these two drugs.

Substance	Route	Signs and Symptoms of Use	Withdrawal Signs and Symptoms	Consequences of Use
Cocaine				

Substance	Route	Signs and Symptoms of Use	Withdrawal Signs and Symptoms	Consequences of Use
Marijuana				

➜ • Click on **Nursing Admission** and read the report.

3. In addition to caffeine, Laura Wilson is abusing two other drugs. These two drugs are

_____ and _____.

4. Explain how these two drugs might affect the health of her baby.

5. The Nursing Admission contains information regarding Laura Wilson's precipitating stressors. Place an X next to the stressors she has identified.

_____ Her parents disapprove of her lifestyle.

_____ She is HIV-positive.

_____ This is an unplanned pregnancy.

_____ She needs to quit "crack."

_____ Her boyfriend is out of town.

6. Select the best coping resource that is available to Laura Wilson at this time.

a. Younger sister
b. Boyfriend
c. Mother and father
d. Roommate

7. Laura Wilson's most frequently used coping mechanisms for dealing with her problems are

_____ and _____.

Exercise 3

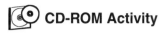 **CD-ROM Activity**

 30 minutes

- Sign in to work at Pacific View Regional Hospital on the Obstetrics Floor for Period of Care 2. (*Note:* If you are already in the virtual hospital from a previous exercise, click on **Leave the Floor** and then **Restart the Program** to get to the sign-in window.)
- From the Patient List, select Laura Wilson (Room 206).
- Click on **Go to Nurses' Station**.
- Click on **206** at the bottom of the screen.
- Click on **Patient Care** and then on **Nurse-Client Interactions**.
- Select and view the video titled **1115: Teaching—Effects of Drug Use**. (*Note:* Check the virtual clock to see whether enough time has elapsed. You can use the fast-forward feature to advance the time by 2-minute intervals if the video is not yet available. Then click on **Patient Care** and **Nurse-Client Interactions** to refresh the screen.)

1. Which of the statements made by Laura Wilson during the interaction best illustrate her lack of understanding regarding substance abuse?

   a. "The baby will help me stay on track."
   b. "It's not like I'm addicted. I can quit anytime."
   c. "It's not like the baby will be addicted."
   d. "I have quit for a month or two."
   e. All except d.

2. Place an X next to the statement(s) that may indicate Laura Wilson's readiness to abstain from drugs.

   _____   "It wasn't a hard decision for me. I am looking forward to this baby."

   _____   "I can go for a while without taking drugs."

   _____   "My mom doesn't believe I can do it."

   _____   "I'll do whatever it takes to keep my baby."

3. What do you believe are the barriers to Laura Wilson's abstinence from drugs?

4. Evaluate the nurse's role in educating Laura Wilson on the effects of drug use.

→ • Click on **MAR**. Verify that you are looking at Laura Wilson's records.
  • Locate the medication ordered for pain.
  • Click on **Return to Room 206** and then on the **Drug** icon in the lower left corner of the screen. Find and review this medication.

5. The medication ordered for Laura Wilson's pain is _____. In this patient's situation, the two most important features of this medication are

_____ and

_____.

6. An important aspect of Laura Wilson's treatment plan will be the teaching plan. Match the patient's education needs to the interventions that will best help her.

Education Needs	**Effective Interventions**
_____ HIV-positive status	a. Well-baby clinic and parental support
_____ Caring for the newborn	b. Community AA-based self-help group and individual motivational and cognitive behavioral approaches
_____ Drug abstinence	
_____ Handling family conflict	c. HIV counselor/HIV clinic
_____ Community resources	d. Discuss with hospital social worker/ discharge planner
	e. Family counseling

7. Relapses are common during a person's recovery. For patients who abuse substances, a key aspect of discharge planning is relapse prevention. The goal for relapse prevention is

_____

_____.

8. Relapse should not be viewed as a total failure because it can result in a renewed and refined effort toward change. Identify and discuss the key elements of relapse prevention strategies the nurse can use with Laura Wilson.

Relapse prevention strategies

9. Community resources will be needed to assist Laura Wilson in her recovery. Select the community resource(s) you think might be helpful to her.

   a. 12-step recovery program
   b. Intensive outpatient program
   c. Relapse prevention group
   d. Individual, group, or family therapy
   e. All of the above

LESSON 11

Crisis and Disaster

Reading Assignment: Crisis and Disaster (Chapter 23)

Patient: Dorothy Grant, Obstetrics Floor, Room 201

Goal: To understand how to provide nursing care for a patient in a health crisis using crisis intervention theory and techniques.

Objectives:

- Define the characteristics and types of crises.
- List factors that limit a person's ability to deal effectively with crises.
- Describe the three types of crises.
- Describe the phases in response to a crisis.
- Define crisis and crisis intervention.
- Identify components in a safety assessment.
- Understand the steps involved in crisis intervention.
- Describe counseling strategies associated with each level of nursing care in crisis intervention.

Exercise 1

Clinical Preparation: Writing Activity

30 minutes

1. Everyone can experience a crisis and either struggle to resolve it or make the necessary

   adjustments to live with it. A _____, caused by a perceived threat or stressful event, is an acute, time-limited occurrence in which a person experiences overwhelming emotional reactions that include tension, helplessness, and disorganization.

2. Many factors may limit a person's ability to problem-solve or cope with stressful life events or situations. Place an X next to all factors that apply.

   _____ Concurrent stressful events with which the person is coping

   _____ Quality and quantity of a person's usual coping skills

   _____ Presence of concurrent medical conditions

   _____ Presence of concurrent psychiatric disorders

   _____ Excessive pain or fatigue

   _____ Presence of unresolved losses

3. Describe three types of crises and give an example of each.

4. When working with a patient in crisis, the nurse's initial task is to promote patient safety.

   That includes assessing the patient's risk for _____ or

   _____.

5. During a crisis, a person's equilibrium may be adversely affected by a lack of one or more balancing factors. Therefore the nurse assesses the patient for three balancing factors that can help an individual during a crisis. They are:

   1.

   2.

   3.

6. Describe four phases in a response to a crisis.

7. _____ is a brief, focused, and time-limited (approximately 6 weeks in length) treatment strategy that focuses on the rapid resolution of an immediate crisis, employing all available resources.

8. Below, explain the steps the nurse would take in providing crisis intervention and list the corresponding crisis intervention components within the step.

Crisis Intervention Step	Crisis Intervention Components
Assessment	
Possible nursing diagnoses	
Outcomes identification	
Planning and implementation	
Evaluation	

9. There are three levels of nursing care in crisis intervention. Match each of the following counseling strategies to its level of nursing care.

Counseling Strategy	**Level of Nursing Care in Crisis Intervention**
_____ Provide support for person who has experienced a severe crisis	a. Primary
_____ Establish interventions during an acute crisis to prevent prolonged anxiety	b. Secondary
_____ Evaluate stressful life events the person is experiencing	c. Tertiary
_____ Ensure the safety of the patient	
_____ Facilitate optimal levels of functioning	
_____ Teach specific coping skills	
_____ Plan environmental changes and make important interpersonal decisions	
_____ Assess the problem, support systems, and coping styles	
_____ Implement critical incident stress debriefing (CISD)	

Exercise 2

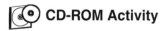 **CD-ROM Activity**

 30 minutes

- Sign in to work at Pacific View Regional Hospital on the Obstetrics Floor for Period of Care 1. (*Note:* If you are already in the virtual hospital from a previous exercise, click on **Leave the Floor** and then **Restart the Program** to get to the sign-in window.)
- From the Patient List, select Dorothy Grant (Room 201).
- Click on **Get Report** and read the shift report.

1. What information in the shift report would alert the nurse that a more thorough psychosocial assessment is needed?

It is important for the nurse to obtain more complete information in caring for Dorothy Grant.

 • Click on **Go to Nurses' Station**.
- Click on **Chart** then on **201** for Dorothy Grant's chart.
- Click on **History and Physical** and review.
- Click on **Nursing Admission** and review.

2. In the History and Physical, what information indicates that Dorothy Grant may be in crisis?

a. Dorothy Grant is 30 weeks pregnant.
b. Her husband beat her and kicked her in the abdomen.
c. Her children are home alone.
d. Her mother was beaten by her father.
e. All of the above.

3. The first step in crisis intervention is assessing the patient in five important areas. In the Nursing Admission, what assessment information did the nurse obtain regarding Dorothy Grant's abuse by her husband? Record your findings below.

Element of Crisis Intervention Assessment	Assessment Data Found
Precipitating event	
Perception of the event	
Support system	
Coping resources	
Coping mechanisms	

4. Given Dorothy Grant's perception of the event and her coping mechanisms, what crisis intervention techniques might work best at this time?

5. Provide at least one example of how the nurse could help Dorothy Grant regain her self-worth.

Child, Older Adult, and Intimate Partner Abuse

∽ **Reading Assignment:** Child, Older Adult, and Intimate Partner Abuse (Chapter 26)

Patient: Dorothy Grant, Obstetrics Floor, Room 201

Goal: To care for a patient who is a survivor of family violence.

Objectives:

- Define family violence.
- Define characteristics common to violent families.
- Describe the three stages in the cycle of violence.
- Understand the differences between myths and realities associated with survivors of abuse.
- Discuss the use of empowerment intervention with women who have been abused.
- Describe strengths and coping strategies of someone who is experiencing abuse or violence.
- Discuss nursing assessment and interventions for a patient experiencing family violence.
- Identify central themes in abusive relationships.
- Understand common barriers to battered spouses leaving the abusive relationship.
- Describe critical elements of discharge planning for someone who is being abused.

Exercise 1

 Clinical Preparation: Writing Activity

 15 minutes

1. Provide a definition of family violence.

2. In terms of comorbidity, the secondary effects of violence are _____,

   _____, and _____ that often last a lifetime.

3. There is a predictable cycle of violence that involves three stages, also described as a process of escalation-deescalation. Match each stage to its characteristics.

   Characteristics   **Stage of Violence Cycle**

   _____ Perpetrator releases built-up tension by   a. Tension-building stage
           brutal and uncontrollable beatings; severe
           injuries may result; both victim and   b. Acute battering stage
           perpetrator are in shock.
                                                           c. Honeymoon stage
   _____ Kind and loving behaviors, expressions
           of remorse, and apologies by the perpetrator;
           victim believes perpetrator and drops any
           legal action.

   _____ Minor incidents such as verbal abuse,
           pushing, and shoving occur; as tension
           escalates, both try to reduce it; perpetrator
           may use alcohol or drugs, which makes
           tension build further.

4. There are several myths regarding survivors of abuse. Describe the reality associated with the myths listed below.

Myth	Reality
Abused spouses can end the violence by leaving their abuser.	
The victim can learn to stop doing things that provoke the violence.	
Being pregnant protects a woman from battering.	
Abused women tacitly accept the abuse by trying to conceal it, not reporting it, or failing to seek help.	

5. Strong negative feelings can cloud a nurse's judgment and interfere with the necessary assessment and interventions. Therefore the attitudes that the nurses bring to these situations shape their responses toward survivors of violence. Place an X next to each true statement.

_____ Nurses may blame survivors if their behavior leading up to the abuse was questionable.

_____ Nurses have difficulty understanding why a battered woman will not leave her abuser.

_____ Nurses may have come from violent environments themselves and identify too closely with the victim.

_____ Nurses may offer advice and sympathy instead of respect.

_____ Nurses may have strong feelings of anger toward the perpetrator.

_____ More nurses have been victimized by violence than has any other work group.

_____ Nurses may want to blame the victim for the problems of abuse.

_____ Nurses who have had clinical experiences with survivors of violence may be less apt to blame than nurses who have not.

6. What is your attitude about domestic violence? How was your attitude shaped?

Exercise 2

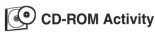 **CD-ROM Activity**

 15 minutes

- Sign in to work at Pacific View Regional Hospital on the Obstetrics Floor for Period of Care 2. (*Note:* If you are already in the virtual hospital from a previous exercise, click on **Leave the Floor** and then **Restart the Program** to get to the sign-in window.)
- From the Patient List, select Dorothy Grant (Room 201).
- Click on **Go to Nurses' Station**.
- Click on **Chart** and then on **201**.
- Click on **Nursing Admission** and review.
- Next, click on **Consultations** and read the Psychiatric Consult and the Social Work Consult.
- Now click on **Mental Health** and read the Psychiatric/Mental Health Assessment, the Depression Inventory, and the Abuse Assessment Screening.

1. Of the five forms that abuse can take within families, place an X next to the forms of abuse Dorothy Grant is experiencing.

    _____ Physical

    _____ Sexual

    _____ Emotional

    _____ Neglect

    _____ Economic

2. Dorothy Grant is in one of the special populations that are vulnerable to abuse. These

    include children, the elderly, the developmentally disabled, and

    _____. The most widespread form of family violence is

    _____.

3. There are general characteristics common to violent families. Below, list the specific characteristics of Dorothy Grant's family that correspond to each of the general characteristics of violent families.

Characteristic of Violent Families	Dorothy Grant's Family
Multigenerational history	
Social isolation	
Use and abuse of power	
Alcohol and drug abuse	

4. What are Dorothy Grant's strengths in dealing with her abusive situation?

5. What are Dorothy Grant's coping strategies in dealing with her abusive relationship?

6. Depression is a common response by women in abusive relationships. According to

   Dorothy Grant's Depression Scale, her level of depression is _____.

Exercise 3

 CD-ROM Activity

 30 minutes

- Sign in to work at Pacific View Regional Hospital on the Obstetrics Floor for Period of Care 2. (*Note:* If you are already in the virtual hospital from a previous exercise, click on **Leave the Floor** and then **Restart the Program** to get to the sign-in window.)
- From the Patient List, select Dorothy Grant (Room 201).
- Click on **Go to Nurses' Station** and then on **201** at the bottom of the screen.
- Click on **Patient Care** and then on **Nurse-Client Interactions**.
- Select and view the video titled **1115: Nurse-Patient Communication**. (*Note:* Check the virtual clock to see whether enough time has elapsed. You can use the fast-forward feature to advance the time by 2-minute intervals if the video is not yet available. Then click on **Patient Care** and **Nurse-Client Interactions** to refresh the screen.)

1. The primary goal of intervention is empowerment, found to be very effective in working with battered women. In the video you just observed, the nurse uses techniques that support this goal when interacting with Dorothy Grant. Below and on the next page, cite specific examples to show how the nurse supports each principle associated with empowerment. (*Hint:* If you are unable to find an example from the nurse's responses, create a response the nurse could use to meet the empowerment goal.)

Principle Associated with Empowerment	Nurse's Response
There is a mutual sharing of knowledge and information	
The nurse strategizes with the survivor	

Principle Associated with Empowerment	Nurse's Response
Survivors are helped to recognize societal influences	
The survivor's competence and experience are respected	

2. The nurse uses other therapeutic responses when interacting with Dorothy Grant. Match each of the following responses to its technique.

Technique	Nurse's Response
_____ Mutual goal sharing	a. "Feeling scared is a perfectly normal reaction."
_____ Focusing	b. "The CNS and the SW work together to identify your immediate needs."
_____ Broad open-ended questions	c. "Right now your first priority is your own well-being and the well-being of your children."
_____ Listening	d. "Would you like to talk about your concerns now? Is there anything I can do to help?"

3. The immediate goal of the nurse in working with Dorothy Grant is to develop trust. In order to develop trust, the nurse must express nonjudgmental listening and psychological support. How did the nurse accomplish (or *not* accomplish) this in the video?

4. What constraints will make it difficult for Dorothy Grant to leave her husband?

   a. She is still in love with her husband.
   b. She lacks housing and financial resources.
   c. Her church affiliation supports marriage.
   d. There is a societal stigma associated with a wife leaving her husband.
   e. Domestic violence reporting is not mandatory in any state.
   f. Her husband is in jail.
   g. Only b and c apply.

5. Dorothy Grant has left her husband twice before and returned. For the battered woman, what do you think is the purpose of this behavior?

6. One of the most frightening realities Dorothy Grant may face in leaving her husband is that

   he might try to _____.

7. Several themes expressed by women in abusive relationships have been identified. Knowing the themes Dorothy Grant is expressing will help the nurse in her assessment and interventions. Identify these below.

Themes of Women Who Have Been in Abusive Relationships	Dorothy Grant's Themes
Lack of relationships outside the home	
Immobility to take action	
Internal feeling of emptiness	
Feeling of being disconnected	

8. Discharge planning will be crucial for Dorothy Grant. Place an X next to all the activities that will be necessary for a successful outcome.

_____   Create a safety planning checklist.

_____   Provide her with hotline phone numbers of other survivors of abuse and violence.

_____   Find a supportive alternate living arrangement for Dorothy Grant and her children.

9. Discuss your own thoughts about Dorothy Grant's current and past responses to the abuse. Do you believe her responses have been more pathological in nature, or do you think she has responded in the typical way a person would react to incredible physical and emotional trauma?

10. Because family violence is a symptom of a family in crisis, what role, if any, do you think family therapy has for Dorothy Grant and her family?

LESSON **13** ————————————————————

Disorders of Children and Adolescents

————————————————————

∽∂ **Reading Assignment:** Disorders of Children and Adolescents (Chapter 28)

Patient: Tiffany Sheldon, Pediatrics Floor, Room 305

Goal: To provide psychiatric nursing care to an adolescent patient.

Objectives:

- Understand the developmental tasks of adolescence.
- Identify key areas to be included when assessing an adolescent patient.
- Explore unhealthy responses seen in adolescence.
- Describe nursing interventions effective in working with adolescents.
- Explore your own issues when working with adolescent patients.
- Evaluate treatment outcomes for an adolescent patient.

Exercise 1

Clinical Preparation: Writing Activity

15 minutes

1. Adolescents have several important tasks to accomplish before transitioning into adulthood. Place an X next to the tasks you think are important for an adolescent to accomplish in order to successfully transition into adulthood.

   _____ Achieving new and more mature relationships with peers of both sexes.

   _____ Preparing for marriage, family life, and career.

   _____ Accepting one's own physical build and using the body effectively.

   _____ Achieving emotional independence from parents and other adults.

2. During an assessment the nurse must include key components specific to the adolescent patient, always checking for high-risk problems. Place an X next to components that would be important to include for this special population.

   _____ Self-concept

   _____ Emotional and physical status

   _____ Social skills and friendships

   _____ Activities of daily living

   _____ Ability to cope with stress and anxiety

   _____ Family life and health

   _____ Suicidal risk

3. Adolescents think and worry about many issues. Typical issues of most adolescents include:

   a. Body image
   b. Identity
   c. Independence
   d. Social role
   e. Sexual behavior
   f. All of the above

4. Body image, identity, and independence are three issues that can produce a variety of healthy and unhealthy responses as the adolescent attempts to cope with the developmental tasks at hand. Match each issue of adolescence with its characteristics.

Adolescent Issue	**Characteristics**
_____ Body image	a. Seen as being free of parental control; seeking out adult situations; may become frightened and overwhelmed in the process.
_____ Identity	
_____ Independence	b. Growth and development vary widely; growth is uneven and sudden; compare self to peers.
	c. Childhood dreams end; become negative and contrary; may feel isolated, lonely, and confused.

Exercise 2

 CD-ROM Activity

 30 minutes

- Sign in to work at Pacific View Regional Hospital on the Pediatrics Floor for Period of Care 3. (*Note:* If you are already in the virtual hospital from a previous exercise, click on **Leave the Floor** and then **Restart the Program** to get to the sign-in window.)
- From the Patient List, select Tiffany Sheldon (Room 305).
- Click on **Go to Nurses' Station**.
- Click on **Chart** and then on **305**.
- Click on **History and Physical** and read.
- Click on **Nursing Admission** and read.
- Click on **Consultations** and read the Psychiatric Consult.

1. In working with adolescents, it is important to distinguish between age-expected behavior and unhealthy coping responses. For each issue listed below and on the next page, identify the age-expected behavior. Then, based on your review of the patient's chart, list Tiffany Sheldon's unhealthy coping responses for each issue.

Issue in Adolescence	Age-Expected Behavior	Tiffany's Unhealthy Response
Body image		

Issue in Adolescence	Age-Expected Behavior	Tiffany's Unhealthy Response
Mood		
Activity		

2. The specific problems of adolescence that make Tiffany Sheldon a high-risk adolescent are:

   a. substance use and truancy.
   b. severe eating disorder and depressed mood.
   c. suicidal and self-injurious.
   d. problems with conduct and violence.
   e. anxiety and sexual promiscuity.

3. When working with adolescents, it is important for the nurse to understand a few basic principles. Place an X next to the statements that best represent the nurse's understanding of these principles in working with Tiffany Sheldon.

   _____ Meet individually with Tiffany to form an alliance and gain her perspective.

   _____ Provide Tiffany with information about healthy and unhealthy adolescent activities.

   _____ Provide Tiffany written health information since she may be too embarrassed to listen to verbal information.

   _____ Educate Tiffany on normal teen behaviors.

   _____ Meet with Tiffany only when her parents are present.

   _____ Help Tiffany build healthy coping skills to deal with stress.

4. In working with Tiffany Sheldon on the psychological aspects of her unhealthy coping responses, discuss the type of therapy suggested in the Psychiatric Consult and give a possible rationale for each suggestion.

5. In thinking about Tiffany Sheldon's problems, what are your own feelings about adolescence that might arise in working with a patient such as this?

6. The nurse must objectively evaluate the nursing care that has been provided to Tiffany and her family. Place an X next to the questions that might be important to ask in determining whether Tiffany and her family have met the treatment goals outlined in the treatment plan.

_____ Were Tiffany's and her parents' concerns addressed?

_____ Has Tiffany's problematic behavior decreased and been replaced with more healthy coping responses?

_____ Have Tiffany's interpersonal relationships improved?

_____ Have Tiffany's activities of daily living become more reasonable in intensity?

_____ Do Tiffany and her family have a better understanding of her problems?

_____ Are Tiffany and her parents satisfied with the progress toward treatment goals?

_____ Is Tiffany at 100% of her normal body weight?

Psychosocial Needs of the Older Adult

———————————————————————————————————————

Reading Assignment: Psychosocial Needs of the Older Adult (Chapter 29)

Patient: Kathryn Doyle, Skilled Nursing Floor, Room 503

Goal: To understand, assess, and care for the elderly patient.

Objectives:

- Identify symptoms of mental illness in the elderly.
- Discuss theories of aging from a variety of perspectives.
- Understand specialized skills of the geropsychiatric nurse.
- Acknowledge biases in working with the elderly patient.
- Perform a comprehensive geriatric assessment.
- Identify common responses that elderly people have in relation to the aging process.
- Plan and coordinate the care for a geriatric patient.
- Know effective treatment strategies to use with the elderly patient and family.
- Identify sources of community aftercare support for the elderly patient and family.

Exercise 1

 Clinical Preparation: Writing Activity

15 minutes

1. Mental illness in the elderly is less likely to be accurately diagnosed because the symptoms

   may be attributed to the _____. This is especially true for

   elderly patients with the diagnoses of _____ and _____.

2. Mental health in late life depends on a number of factors. Which of the following factors
   might affect the mental health of the elderly?

   a. Physiological and psychological status
   b. Economic resources
   c. Social support systems
   d. Personality
   e. Lifestyle
   f. All of the above

3. Ageism is an important issue that affects how a nurse will care for the elderly patient.
   Define ageism and discuss its implications for health care delivery.

4. Positive attitudes toward elderly patients and their care must be developed in nursing education programs. To accomplish this, nursing education programs need to include:
   a. Information about the aging process
   b. Discussion of the attitudes in working with the elderly
   c. Exploration of nurse-patient interactions
   d. Development of methods for nursing students to become sensitive to the needs of the elderly
   e. Discussion of the increased prevalence of elderly patients in hospital beds
   f. Providing respect to older patients and appreciating their wisdom and life experience.
   g. All except e

5. Describe the specialized nursing skills necessary to care for the elderly patient.

6. Discuss possible biases you may have in working with the elderly.

Exercise 2

 CD-ROM Activity

 45 minutes

- Sign in to work at Pacific View Regional Hospital on the Skilled Nursing Floor for Period of Care 2. (*Note:* If you are already in the virtual hospital from a previous exercise, click on **Leave the Floor** and then **Restart the Program** to get to the sign-in window.)
- From the Patient List, select Kathryn Doyle (Room 503).
- Click **Go to Nurses' Station**.
- Click on **Chart** and then on **503**.
- Click on **Nursing Admission** and read this record.
- Click on **History and Physical** and read.
- Next, click on **Consultations** and read the Psychiatric Clinical Nurse Specialist Consult.

1. The four Ds of a comprehensive geriatric assessment are delirium, dementia, depression, and delusions. According to the medical record, Kathryn Doyle has depression. Depression is often confused with dementia and is not always recognized. Therefore the nurse needs to be familiar with the symptoms of later-life depression. What symptoms is Kathryn Doyle experiencing that are consistent with later-life depression?

2. In addition to her depression, Kathryn Doyle also seems to be experiencing anxiety. Which of these statements are true regarding anxiety in the elderly?

   _____ Comorbid anxiety and depression are common in the elderly.

   _____ All types of anxiety combined are more prevalent than depression in the elderly.

   _____ Untreated anxiety can contribute to sleep problems, cognitive impairments, and decreased quality of life.

   _____ Anxiety does not affect the family.

   _____ Antianxiety medications may also decrease depression.

3. Besides interviewing the geriatric patient and completing a mental status, there are other key components of the geropsychiatric nursing assessment. For each component listed below and on the next page, include the key elements to be considered. Then list data specific to Kathryn Doyle based on your review of her chart.

Component	Key Elements	Assessment of Kathryn Doyle
Behavioral responses		
Functional abilities		
Physiological responses		

Component	Key Elements	Assessment of Kathryn Doyle
Social support		

 • Click on **Return to Nurses' Station** and then on **503** at the bottom of the screen.
- Inside the patient's room, click on **Patient Care** and then on **Nurse-Client Interactions**.
- Select and view the video titled **1150: Assessment—Depression**. (*Note:* Check the virtual clock to see whether enough time has elapsed. You can use the fast-forward feature to advance the time by 2-minute intervals if the video is not yet available. Then click on **Patient Care** and **Nurse-Client Interactions** to refresh the screen.)

4. Depression and sadness are sometimes viewed as a normal part of aging. Kathryn Doyle's response to life events that have occurred over the past 9 months has resulted in a disturbance in her mood. Place an X next to each correct statement as it pertains to Kathryn Doyle's diagnosis of depression.

_____ The death of her husband has compounded the cumulative losses she has experienced.

_____ She is experiencing prolonged mourning over the loss of her husband.

_____ She demonstrates a loss of interest in her friends and her usual activities.

_____ She is experiencing a loss of independence as a result of her hip fracture.

_____ She is experiencing symptoms of loss of appetite and resulting weight loss.

_____ She has symptoms of fatigue and apathy.

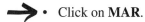 • Click on **MAR**.
• Review Kathryn Doyle's medication list.

5. Does Kathryn Doyle have medication ordered to treat her depression? Discuss the role of medication to treat depression in the elderly.

6. Based on the nurse's assessment, Kathryn Doyle has other affective, somatic, stress, and behavioral responses common to the elderly. Complete the table below and on the next page outlining Kathryn Doyle's specific issues associated with these common reactions.

Type of Response	Issues Involved with Kathryn Doyle's Response
Situational low self-esteem	
Imbalanced nutrition	
Relocation stress syndrome	

Type of Response	Issues Involved with Kathryn Doyle's Response
Social isolation	

Let's jump ahead in virtual time to observe a later interaction between the nurse and Kathryn Doyle.

- Click on **Return to Room 503**.
- Click on **Leave the Floor** and then on **Restart the Program**.
- Sign in to work on the Skilled Nursing Floor, this time for Period of Care 3.
- From the Patient List, select Kathryn Doyle (Room 503).
- Click on **Go to Nurses' Station**.
- Click on **503** at the bottom of the screen.
- Click on **Patient Care** and then on **Nurse-Client Interactions**.
- Select and view the video titled **1505: Assessment—Elder Abuse**. (*Note:* Check the virtual clock to see whether enough time has elapsed. You can use the fast-forward feature to advance the time by 2-minute intervals if the video is not yet available. Then click on **Patient Care** and **Nurse-Client Interactions** to refresh the screen.)

7. Elder neglect and abuse have become more common in our society as elderly people no longer have the status of respect they once had through their extended families. Serving as Kathryn Doyle's advocate, the nurse must be alert for signs of elder neglect, abuse, or exploitation. What are the signs that Kathryn Doyle is being neglected, exploited, or abused?

8. During the family conference, the issue of theft will be addressed. Another concern that will need to be discussed is Kathryn Doyle continuing to live in her son's home post hip fracture. For the current living arrangement to work, the environment must include several basic characteristics therapeutic for elderly patients. Place an X next to the critical elements you think should be included in Kathryn Doyle's home environment.

_____ Sense of calm and quiet

_____ Structured routine, usual for her lifestyle

_____ Consistent physical layout

_____ Activities that produce cognitive stimulation

_____ Safe environment

_____ Personal items that provide familiarity and a sense of security

_____ Focus on her strengths and abilities

9. Today, most elderly people are cared for in the home. What topics should the nurse include in family education and support sessions that would be critical to Kathryn Doyle's recovery and future?

10. Aftercare for elderly patients is often necessary for a successful treatment outcome. After discharge, what agency support do you think Kathryn Doyle's son will need in the care of his mother in the home?

LESSON 15 ——————————————————

Integrative Care

————————————————————————————

👓 **Reading Assignment:** Integrative Care (Chapter 36)

Patient: Kelly Brady, Obstetrics Floor, Room 203

Goal: To provide nursing care to a patient with anxiety and depression, utilizing complementary and alternative treatments and approaches.

Objectives:

• Define integrative care.
• Define complementary and alternative medicine (CAM) and treatments.
• Discuss the trend toward the use of complementary and alternative treatments.
• List the types of complementary and alternative treatments and approaches.
• Refer patients to reliable resources on CAMs.
• Discuss complementary and alternative treatments for a patient with depression and anxiety.

Exercise 1

 Clinical Preparation: Writing Activity

30 minutes

1. Combining conventional medical care with complementary and alternative medicine using a holistic approach is called _____ care.

2. _____ therapy refers to substitute therapies for conventional therapies.

   _____ therapy refers to therapies used in conjunction with conventional therapies. Together these are called _____, or

   _____ for short.

3. It is important for the nurse to become familiar with complementary and alternative therapies. Place an X next to each statement that helps to explain why this may be true.

   _____ Approximately 50% of people in the United States use some form of CAM.

   _____ Some CAMs may interfere with conventional treatments.

   _____ Nurses can appreciate the holistic nature of combining CAM with traditional medicine.

   _____ Some people think treatments that are called "natural" are harmless.

   _____ Many people who use CAMs do not check with their conventional practitioners.

4. With readily available medical information, knowledgeable consumers are questioning the traditional practice of conventional medicine and turning to complementary and alternative therapies and treatments for a variety of disorders. Select the statements that best explain this trend.

   a. CAM practitioners spend more time with and learn more about their patients.
   b. Patients want to find effective therapeutic approaches that carry less risk than medications.
   c. Patients are tired of rushed office visits where conventional practitioners are too busy to listen to their problems.
   d. Patients want to find less expensive alternatives to high-cost conventional care.
   e. Patients want to be actively engaged in their care.
   f. All of the above.

5. According to the National Center for Complementary and Alternative Medicine (NCCAM), integrative care is grouped into four domains. Provide at least one example of a complementary and/or alternative therapy and treatment for each domain below.

Domain	Examples
Mind-body interventions	
Biologically based therapies	
Manipulative practices	
Energy therapies	

6. The nurse must be able to direct patients to reliable and professional information on CAMs. One organization that disseminates information on CAM to practitioners and the public is

the _____, a branch of the National Institutes of Health (NIH). Both practitioners and the public may visit http://nccam.nih.gov for more information.

7. In thinking about the reasons more people are turning to complementary and alternative medicine, what steps could the nurse take to demonstrate his or her willingness to work closely with patients who may also be using CAMs?

Exercise 2

 CD-ROM Activity

 30 minutes

- Sign in to work at Pacific View Regional Hospital on the Obstetrics Floor for Period of Care 3. (*Note:* If you are already in the virtual hospital from a previous exercise, click on **Leave the Floor** and then **Restart the Program** to get to the sign-in window.)
- From the Patient List, select Kelly Brady (Room 203).
- Click on **Go to Nurses' Station**.
- Click on **Chart** and then on **203**.
- Click on **Nursing Admission** and review.

1. The nurse asks two questions in the admission assessment that refer to Kelly Brady's use of complementary/alternative therapies and spiritual and cultural practices. What are these two questions, and how did the patient answer them?

 • Now click on **Consultations** and review the Psychiatric Consult.

2. Kelly Brady has multiple stressors in her life creating anxiety and depression. Select the stressors with which she is struggling.

   a. Mother diagnosed with cancer and parents out of town for treatment
   b. Husband's job not stable; moving to a more expensive home
   c. Has a high-stress job; her work performance has decreased
   d. Potential health problems of her baby due to preeclampsia and premature delivery
   e. All of the above

3. Kelly Brady has several conventional treatments recommended. Place an X next to each conventional treatment listed in the Psychiatric Consult plan.

_____ Paroxetine 20 mg post C-section

_____ Cognitive, couples, and family therapy

_____ Education regarding depression

_____ Anxiety-reduction techniques

➡ • Still in the chart, click on **Mental Health**. Review the Psychiatric/Mental Health Assessment.

4. Kelly Brady has provided the nurse with information regarding how she has been coping with stress. Select the methods the patient has used to try to deal with her stress.

   a. Cries and becomes irritable
   b. Gets extra sleep
   c. Plays music and cooks
   d. Tries to go to gym or plays golf with husband on weekends
   e. Does both b and c

5. When the nurse asks her what she wants to change, Kelly Brady states that she wants better

   _____ in her life between work and home. The nurse then asks her

   whether she uses any CAMs, and her reply is that she has practiced _____
   in the past.

6. There are several integrative approaches to the treatment of anxiety and depression. From the CAM therapies listed in your text, list five approaches you believe may be beneficial in treating both anxiety and depression. Which of these approaches are found in Kelly Brady's treatment plan?

7. According to Kelly Brady's Nursing Admission, she reads the Bible and prays and has arranged for her pastor to visit her in the hospital. Discuss the benefits of prayer as a complementary therapy.

8. In reviewing Kelly Brady's past attempts to control her anxiety and depression, what other complementary treatments or therapies would you recommend for her?